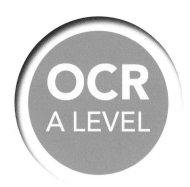

OCR
A LEVEL

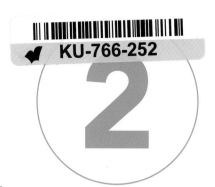

2

PE
FOR A LEVEL

John Honeybourne
Sarah Powell

An OCR endorsed textbook

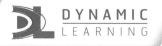

DYNAMIC LEARNING

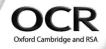

OCR
Oxford Cambridge and RSA

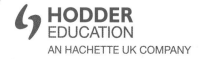

HODDER
EDUCATION
AN HACHETTE UK COMPANY

Hachette UK's policy is to use papers that are natural, renewable and recyclable products and made from wood grown in sustainable forests. The logging and manufacturing processes are expected to conform to the environmental regulations of the country of origin.

Orders: please contact Bookpoint Ltd, 130 Park Drive, Milton Park, Abingdon, Oxon OX14 4SE. Telephone: (44) 01235 827720. Fax: (44) 01235 400454. Email education@bookpoint.co.uk Lines are open from 9 a.m. to 5 p.m., Monday to Saturday, with a 24-hour message answering service. You can also order through our website: www.hoddereducation.co.uk

ISBN: 978 1 4718 5174 2

© John Honeybourne and Sarah Powell 2016

First published in 2016 by

Hodder Education,

An Hachette UK Company

Carmelite House

50 Victoria Embankment

London EC4Y 0DZ

www.hoddereducation.co.uk

Impression number   10 9 8 7 6 5 4 3

Year   2020 2019 2018 2017

Cover photo © jocic/Thinkstock/iStockphoto/Getty Images

Typeset in India

Printed in Italy

A catalogue record for this title is available from the British Library.

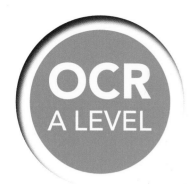

OCR
A LEVEL

2

PE
FOR A LEVEL

Contents

Acknowledgements

The Publishers would like to thank the following for permission to reproduce copyright material.

p. 29, Table 1.2.3: reproduced with permission from Wolters Kluwer, from Wenger, C.B. and Hardy, J.D. (1990) 'Temperature regulation and exposure to heat and cold', in Lehmann, J.F. (ed.) *Therapeutic Heat and Cold*, 4th edition, Baltimore, MD: Williams & Wilkins, pp. 150–178; p. 124, Figure 5.1.4: reproduced with permission from Human Kinetics, from Roberts, G.C. and Pascuzzi, D. (1979) 'Causal attributions in sport: some theoretical implications', *Journal of Sports Psychology*, 1: 203–211.

Photo credits

pp. 1 and 10 (far right): © EMMANUEL DUNAND/AFP/Getty Images; p. 7: © ginasanders/123RF; p. 10 (far left): © Ross Land/Getty Images; p. 10 (middle left): © berc/Fotolia; p. 10 (middle right): © Christophe Schmid/Fotolia; p. 11: © Mike Hewitt/Getty Images; p. 14 (top): © BSIP SA/Alamy Stock Photo; p. 14 (bottom): © Maitree Laipitaksin/123RF; p. 26: © James Brunker/Alamy Stock Photo; p. 31: © Alex Goodlett/Getty Images; pp. 33 and 58: © Matthew Stockman/Getty Images; p. 35: © Peter G. Aiken/Getty Images; p. 37: © Lance King/Getty Images Sport/Getty Images; p. 38: © Powered by Light/Alan Spencer/Alamy Stock Photo; p. 39: © Doug Pensinger/Getty Images Sport/Getty Images; p. 40: © Jae C. Hong/AP/Press Association Images; p. 47: © David Rogers/Getty Images; p. 48: © Scott Heavey/Getty Images; p. 53: © Bupa UK, PRICE info graphic, http://www.bupa.co.uk/health-information, 2016; p. 54: © Catherine Ivill – AMA/Getty Images; p. 55: © David Rogers/Getty Images; p. 57: © Miguel A. Muñoz Pellicer/Alamy Stock Photo; p. 60: © David Hallett/Getty Images; p. 61: © Andre Ferreira/Icon Sport/Getty Images; p. 62 (left): © BSIP SA/Alamy Stock Photo; p. 62 (right): © Clynt Garnham Medical/Alamy Stock Photo; p. 63: © John Peters/Manchester United via Getty Images; p. 65: © Harry How/Getty Images; p. 66: © Alberto Tao/AP/Press Association Images; pp. 69 and 85: © CHRISTOF STACHE/Getty Images; p. 70: © AGF Srl/Alamy Stock Photo; p. 78 (left): © dpa picture alliance archive/Alamy Stock Photo; p. 78 (right): © OLIVIER MORIN/AFP/Getty Images; p. 81: © Tom Jenkins/Getty Images; p. 83 (left): © Design Pics Inc/Alamy Stock Photo; p. 83 (middle): © Jamie Squire/Getty Images Europe/Getty Images; p. 83 (right): © Michael Gray/123RF; p. 88: © Al Bello/Allsport/Getty Images; p. 90: © ZUMA Press, Inc./Alamy Stock Photo; p. 94: © Adam Pretty/Getty Images Sport/Getty Images; p. 95: © European Sports Photographic Agency/Alamy Stock Photo; p. 96 (top): © Alex Livesey/Getty Images; p. 96 (bottom): © Shariff Che'Lah/123RF; p. 98: © warrengoldswain/123RF; p. 104: © Clive Mason/Getty Images; p. 108: © Victor Decolongon/Getty Images; pp. 111 and 117: © Mike Hewitt/Getty Images; p. 114: © lightpoet/123RF; p. 118: © Action Plus Sports Images/Alamy Stock Photo; pp. 121 and 129: © Wavebreak Media Ltd/123RF; p. 122: © Cathy Yeulet/123RF; p. 134: © Paul Marriott/Alamy Stock Photo; p. 142: © Jessmine/Fotolia; p. 143: © anikasalsera/123RF; p. 145: © epa european pressphoto agency b.v./Alamy Stock Photo; p. 147: © wareham.nl (sport)/Alamy Stock Photo; p. 150: © dmbaker/123RF; p. 154: © Sport In Pictures/Alamy Stock Photo; pp. 157 and 188: © Helene Wiesenhaan/Getty Images Sport/Getty Images; p. 161: © stokkete/Fotolia; p. 162: © Oleksandr Prykhodko/Alamy Stock Photo; p. 164: © epa european pressphoto agency b.v./Alamy Stock Photo; p. 167: © Ian Horrocks/Sunderland AFC/Getty Images; p. 169: © Anadolu Agency/Getty Images; p. 171: © roibu/Alamy Stock Photo; p. 172: © Paul Baldesare/Alamy Stock Photo; p. 176: © Jemal Countess/WireImage/Getty Images; p. 178: © Michael Steele/Getty Images; p. 179: © Brandon Griffiths/Alamy Stock Photo; p. 181: © Martin Rose/Bongarts/Getty Images; p. 187: © Sport In Pictures/Alamy Stock Photo; p. 190: © Action Plus Sports Images/Alamy Stock Photo; p. 191 (top): © Michael Buddle/Alamy Stock Photo; p. 191 (bottom): Courtesy of English Institute of Sport; p. 199: © mezzotint/Fotolia; p. 200: © Hans Deryk/AP/Press Association Images; p. 202: © maridav/123RF; p. 203: © Action Plus Sports Images/Alamy Stock Photo; p. 204: © Action Plus Sports Images/Alamy Stock Photo; p. 206: © Photodisc/Getty Images.

Introduction

This OCR-endorsed textbook is designed specifically to cover the specification content for year two of the OCR A Level Physical Education qualification (H555). Each part in the book covers a different main topic area of the OCR specification and each chapter explores in more detail the specification content, along with material that will fully develop each candidate's understanding of each topic area. Year one of the A Level course is covered in OCR PE for A Level Book 1.

The demands of each examination question paper are recognised by the book, including in-depth treatment of each aspect of the specification, enabling candidates to write with the required depth of analysis, including being able to respond effectively to the examinations' extended questions. The book includes extension material to stretch and challenge candidates and to give context to the theoretical principles covered.

Specification coverage

- **Part 1** of this book covers the year two topics for **Applied anatomy and physiology**. It covers Energy for exercise and Environmental effects on body systems. *The other topics in this area are covered in OCR PE for A Level Book 1.*

- **Part 2** of this book covers the year two topics for **Exercise physiology**. It covers Injury prevention and the rehabilitation of injury. *The other topics in this area are covered in OCR PE for A Level Book 1.*

- **Part 3** of this book covers the year two topics for **Biomechanics**. It covers Linear motion, Angular motion, and Fluid mechanics and projectile motion. *The other topics in this area are covered in OCR PE for A Level Book 1.*

- **Part 4** of this book covers the year two content for **Skill acquisition**. It covers Memory models. *The other topics in this area are covered in OCR PE for A Level Book 1*

- **Part 5** of this book covers the year two content for **Sports psychology**. It covers Attribution in sport, Confidence and self-efficacy in sports performance, Leadership in sport, and Stress management to optimise performance. *The other topics in this area are covered in OCR PE for A Level Book 1.*

- **Part 6** of this book covers the complete specification for **Contemporary issues in physical activity and sport** for A Level.

Summary of specification coverage

A Level specification	Covered in Book 1	Covered in Book 2	A Level exam paper
Applied anatomy and physiology	✓ Skeletal and muscular systems ✓ Cardiovascular and respiratory systems	✓ Energy for exercise ✓ Environmental effects on body systems	1
Exercise physiology	✓ Diet and nutrition and their effect on physical activity and performance ✓ Preparation and training methods in relation to improving and maintaining physical activity and performance	✓ Injury prevention and the rehabilitation of injury	1
Biomechanics	✓ Biomechanical principles, levers and the use of technology	✓ Linear motion, angular motion, fluid mechanics and projectile motion	1
Skill acquisition	✓ Classification of skills ✓ Types and methods of practice ✓ Transfer of skills ✓ Principles and theories of learning movement skills ✓ Stages of learning ✓ Guidance ✓ Feedback	✓ Memory models	2
Sports psychology	✓ Individual differences ✓ Group and team dynamics in sport ✓ Goal setting in sports performance	✓ Attribution ✓ Confidence and self-efficacy in sports ✓ Leadership in sport ✓ Stress management to optimise performance	2
Sport and society	✓ Emergence and evolution of modern sport ✓ Global sporting events	All topics covered in Book 1	3
Contemporary issues in physical activity and sport	All topics covered in Book 2	✓ Ethics and deviance in sport ✓ Commercialisation and media ✓ Routes to sporting excellence in the UK ✓ Modern technology in sport – its impact on elite-level sport, participation, fair outcomes and entertainment	3

How to use this book

Understanding the specification
Outline of the main ways the content is related to the specification.

IN THE NEWS
References to contemporary real-life events designed to demonstrate the importance of PE to the world around us.

Key terms
Short definitions of key vocabulary.

Extend your knowledge
Extension material for each chapter that might go slightly beyond the specification but gives extra information for possible use in extended answers.

RESEARCH IN FOCUS
Extracts offering an insight into interesting and relevant contemporary research.

Evaluation
Key tips and information for evaluation of key areas.

Activities
Short tasks and activities to help reinforce learning.

Study hints
Handy tips for studying PE.

Summary
Summary of key points of each chapter.

Check your understanding
Short, knowledge-based questions to help you check you have understood different topics.

Practice questions
Questions designed to offer study practice.

The authors

The authors have been experienced A Level Physical Education teachers themselves, are passionate about their subject and are well qualified in their subject expertise to ensure that this textbook is as relevant and supportive as it can be for this A Level Physical Education qualification. It is written in a style to both engage and inform every candidate whatever their academic ability. The authors hope that the comprehensive coverage of the specification, along with a readable style that applies theory to practice throughout the book, will furnish each OCR A Level Physical Education candidate with all the material necessary to be able to answer A Level examination questions.

Acknowledgements

The authors would like to thank their respective families for their support during the challenging but rewarding writing process.

John Honeybourne BEd; Adv Dip Ed; MA

Dr Sarah Powell BSc; MEd; PhD

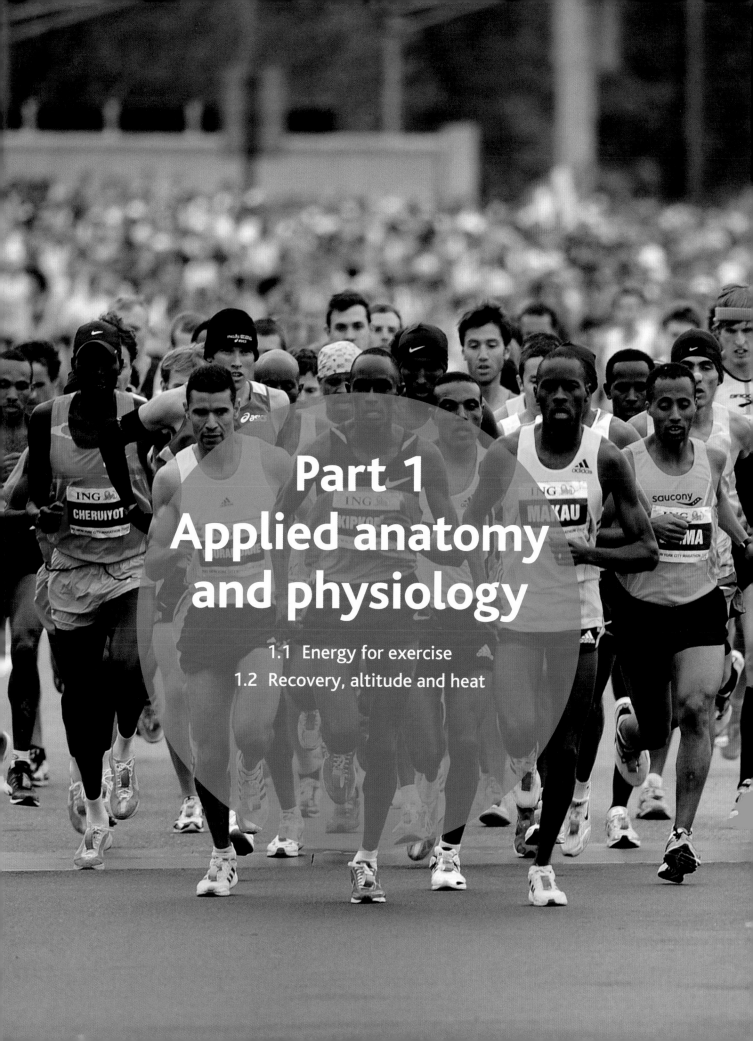

Part 1
Applied anatomy and physiology

1.1 Energy for exercise
1.2 Recovery, altitude and heat

1.1 Energy for exercise

Understanding the specification

By the end of this chapter you should be able to demonstrate knowledge and understanding of the role of adenosine triphosphate (ATP) and its resynthesis during exercise of differing intensities and durations through the three energy systems:

- ATP's key role as an energy currency
- ATP's resynthesis providing energy for exercise
- ATP-PC system
- glycolytic system
- aerobic system
- the energy continuum.

Key terms

Metabolism: the chemical processes that occur within a cell to maintain life. Some substances are broken down to provide energy while others are resynthesised to store energy.

Adenosine triphosphate (ATP): a high-energy compound which is the only immediately available source of energy for muscular contraction.

Enzyme: biological catalyst which increases the speed of chemical reactions.

ATPase: an enzyme which catalyses the breakdown of ATP.

Exothermic reaction: a chemical reaction which releases energy.

Adenosine diphosphate (ADP): a compound formed by the removal of a phosphate bond from ATP (ATP → ADP + P + energy).

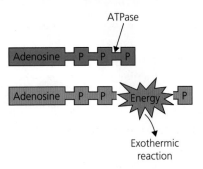

▲ Figure 1.1.1 The release of energy from ATP

Anatomy and physiology is the study of structures and how they function in the human body. To date you have considered the skeletal, muscular, cardiovascular and respiratory systems and how they function to perform physical activity. Applied anatomy and physiology extends further to consider how these systems are provided with the energy required to perform physical activities of varying intensities and durations, and how these systems recover and cope in difficult environmental conditions.

Energy for exercise

Energy is the capacity to perform work and can exist in chemical, potential and kinetic forms. Chemical energy held in the food we eat can be stored as potential energy in the body tissues and converted into kinetic (movement) energy as we contract our muscles. Maximising this process is essential to improve training and performance.

Adenosine triphosphate

The food we eat can be stored in the body as amino acids, triglycerides and glycogen ready to be used as fuel for energy production (see Book 1, Chapter 2.1). When these fuels are **metabolised** they are converted into a compound known as **adenosine triphosphate (ATP)**, the universal energy currency of the human body. When ATP is broken down, energy is provided for cellular processes such as digestion, nerve transmission and muscular contraction.

ATP breakdown

For the exercising body, ATP is stored in the muscle cell and is the only immediately available source of energy for muscular contraction. It is made up of one adenosine and three phosphates held together by bonds of chemical energy. To extract the energy from ATP, the **enzyme ATPase** is released, which stimulates the final high-energy bond to be broken. This **exothermic reaction** releases energy for muscular contraction and leaves **adenosine diphosphate (ADP)** and a single phosphate (P).

ATP resynthesis

The store of ATP in the muscle cell is exhausted quickly, lasting only 2–3 seconds: several powerful contractions or several seconds of sprinting. In order to continue exercising, ATP must be constantly resynthesised or rebuilt. To do this an **endothermic reaction** occurs where energy from the surrounding area is absorbed to rebuild the high-energy bond between ADP and a single phosphate (P). The energy required is provided by one of three energy systems which break down the food fuels stored around the body.

> **Key term**
>
> **Endothermic reaction:** a chemical reaction which absorbs energy.

> **Activity**
>
> Fill in the blanks in the following paragraph:
> ATP is the only immediately available source of _____ for muscular contraction. The enzyme _____ catalyses ATP breakdown to release energy in an exothermic reaction leaving ADP and P. ATP stores in the muscle cell will last around _____ seconds only and must be _____ to continue exercising. In an _____ reaction energy is absorbed from the surrounding area to restore the high-energy bond between the ADP and P resynthesising ATP.

> **Evaluation**
>
> To summarise:
> - Breakdown of ATP:
>   ATP → ADP + P + energy (exothermic reaction)
> - Resynthesis of ATP:
>   ADP + P + energy → ATP (endothermic reaction)

Energy systems

There are three energy systems which break down food fuels to provide the energy for ATP resynthesis:

- ATP-PC system
- glycolytic system
- aerobic system.

At any one time, depending on the intensity and duration of the activity, one energy system will dominate to maintain ATP resynthesis. ATP will then be continuously broken down to provide the energy for muscular contraction for the duration of the activity. If ATP fails to be resynthesised, there will be no energy released for muscular contraction and fatigue will quickly set in.

ATP-PC system

The ATP-PC system kicks in during very high-intensity activity after the first two seconds of intense activity depletes the original ATP stores. ATP levels fall dramatically and ADP and P levels rise. This triggers the release of **creatine kinase**, an enzyme which catalyses the breakdown of the immediately available fuel **phosphocreatine** (PC).

PC (also known as creatine phosphate) is made up of creatine with a high-energy phosphate bond and is stored on site in the muscle cells. Easily accessed PC is a simple structure broken down **anaerobically** in the **sarcoplasm**. The high-energy bond between the creatine and phosphate is broken, releasing energy for ATP resynthesis. For every one **mole** of PC broken down, one mole of ATP can be resynthesised.

This forms a **coupled reaction** whereby the breakdown of PC releases a free phosphate and energy which can then be used to resynthesise ATP. This process happens very quickly as both compounds are simple structures providing energy for very high-intensity activities such as the 60 m and 100 m sprints, throws and jumps in athletics, a gymnastic vault, a sprint up the wing in rugby or a short corner in hockey. However, PC stores are small and quickly exhausted after approximately eight seconds.

> **Key terms**
>
> **Creatine kinase:** an enzyme which catalyses the breakdown of phosphocreatine (PC).
> **Phosphocreatine:** a high-energy compound stored in the muscle cell and broken down for ATP resynthesis.
> **Anaerobic:** without the presence of oxygen.
> **Sarcoplasm:** the cytoplasm or fluid within the muscle cell which holds stores of PC, glycogen and myoglobin.
> **Mole:** a unit of substance quantity.
> **Coupled reaction:** where the products of one reaction are used in another reaction.

Extend your knowledge

To improve the efficiency of the ATP-PC system, anaerobic high-intensity training should be used. Maximal and explosive strength training will increase muscle mass, which boosts the storage capacity for ATP and PC. A performer can supplement creatine and load phosphates in addition to a high-protein diet (for example, lean meat) to maximise the body's stores, of PC. Combining the correct training and diet will maximise the fuel stores, increase the duration of the ATP-PC system, and delay fatigue. This will enable an increased quantity and quality of training.

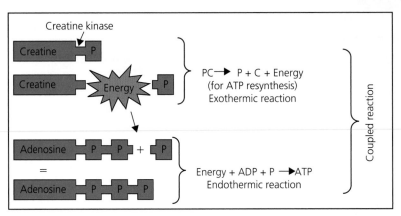

▲ Figure 1.1.2 The coupled reaction of PC breakdown and ATP resynthesis

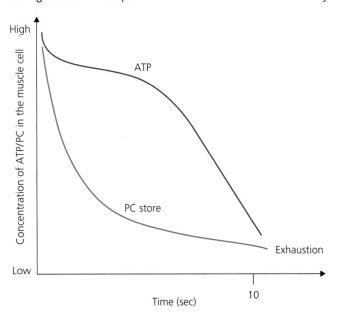

ATP levels remain high as PC levels decline rapidly as the PC stores are broken down to provide the energy to resynthesise ATP. Around six seconds, PC stores start to deplete and ATP resynthesis declines. At ten seconds, PC and ATP stores become exhausted.

▲ Figure 1.1.3 The relative concentration of ATP and PC stores in the muscle cell over ten seconds of exhaustive work

Study hint

Remember the energy released from food fuels such as PC is not used to contract the muscles but to resynthesise ATP. ATP is then broken down to release the energy for muscular contraction.

▼ Table 1.1.1 The key descriptors, strengths and weaknesses of the ATP-PC system

Type of reaction	Anaerobic (without the presence of oxygen)
Site of reaction	Sarcoplasm
Food fuel used	Phosphocreatine (PC)
Controlling enzyme	Creatine kinase
ATP yield	1 mole of PC yields 1 mole of ATP (1:1)
Specific stages	PC → P + C + energy (exothermic) Energy + P + ADP → ATP (endothermic)
By-products	None
Intensity of activity	Very high intensity
Duration of system	2–10 seconds
Strengths	No delay for oxygen PC readily available in the muscle cell Simple and rapid breakdown of PC and resynthesis of ATP Provides energy for very high-intensity activities No fatiguing by-products and simple compounds aid fast recovery
Weaknesses	Low ATP yield and small PC stores lead to rapid fatigue after 8–10 seconds

Glycolytic system

The glycolytic system kicks in during high-intensity activity after the first ten seconds of intense activity exhausts PC stores and ATP levels fall. ADP and P levels rise again and trigger the release of **phosphofructokinase (PFK)**, an enzyme which catalyses the breakdown of the next available fuel: glucose. Glucose is an energy-rich molecule ($C_6H_{12}O_6$) circulating in the blood stream. If glucose levels dip, glycogen phosphorylase (GPP), an enzyme which catalyses the breakdown of stored glycogen (in the muscles and liver), is released, converting glycogen into glucose to maintain its concentration in the blood stream.

Glucose is easily accessed as a fuel, broken down to extract energy for continued ATP resynthesis in the sarcoplasm. The breakdown of glucose in the absence of oxygen is through a process called **anaerobic glycolysis** and results in the production of pyruvic acid. For every one mole of glucose broken down there is a net gain of two moles of ATP. This provides energy for high-intensity activities such as the 200–400 m track events, 100 m freestyle, a counter attack in football or distancing from the pack in a marathon. Glycolytic ATP resynthesis will continue for around three minutes, although its efficiency peaks at one minute and then slowly decreases. At this high intensity oxygen is not available to continue the energy extraction from pyruvic acid and **lactate dehydrogenase (LDH)** is released. LDH is an enzyme which catalyses the conversion of pyruvic acid into lactic acid, which accumulates and slows ATP resynthesis.

Anaerobic glycolysis frees only around 5 per cent of the potential energy held in the glucose molecule and as lactic acid levels rise, the pH in the muscle cells decreases (or acidity increases). This inhibits enzyme activity, preventing further breakdown of fuel and ATP resynthesis, causing local muscular fatigue. The point at which blood lactate levels significantly rise is known as **OBLA** (the onset of blood lactate accumulation) and occurs on average around 4 mmol/l.

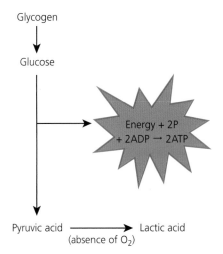

▲ Figure 1.1.4 The key stages of the glycolytic system

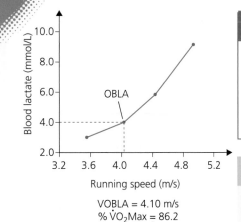

VOBLA = 4.10 m/s
% $\dot{V}O_2$Max = 86.2

▲ Figure 1.1.5 The point at which a national under-19 squash player hits OBLA during a progressive intensity running test

Extend your knowledge

As lactic acid accumulates, hydrogen ions disassociate, leaving lactate. The hydrogen ions are responsible for the acidity and feelings of pain as nerve signals are blocked and exercising limbs become 'heavy'.

Key term

Buffering capacity: the ability of hydrogen carbonate ions (buffers) to neutralise the effects of lactic acid in the blood stream.

Study hint

Using the acronyms for known enzymes in exams is common practice—for example, PFK is perfectly acceptable for phosphofructokinase.

Study hint

Pyruvic acid and lactic acid can also be termed pyruvate and lactate.

Evaluation

To summarise:
- Breakdown of glucose: Glucose → pyruvic acid + energy
- Lactic acid production: Pyruvic acid → lactic acid
- Resynthesis of ATP: Energy + 2P + 2ADP → 2ATP
- Breakdown of ATP: ATP → ADP + P + energy for muscular contraction

Extend your knowledge

To improve the efficiency of the glycolytic system, a combination of high-intensity anaerobic training and aerobic training close to the anaerobic threshold can be performed. This will improve strength endurance, **buffering capacity**, removal of lactic acid and recovery rates. A performer can use glucose and bicarbonate supplements and pre- and post-event meals to maximise the body's stores of glycogen and buffering capacity. Combining the correct training and diet will maximise fuel stores and minimise lactic acid accumulation, delaying OBLA and the early onset of fatigue.

▼ Table 1.1.2 The key descriptors, strengths and weaknesses of the glycolytic system

Type of reaction	Anaerobic (without the presence of oxygen)
Site of reaction	Sarcoplasm
Food fuel used	Glycogen/glucose
Controlling enzyme	GPP, PFK and LDH
ATP yield	1 mole of glycogen yields 2 moles of ATP (1:2)
Specific stages	Anaerobic glycolysis: glycogen/glucose → pyruvic acid + energy Lactate pathway: pyruvic acid → lactic acid Energy + 2P + 2ADP → 2ATP (endothermic)
By-products	Lactic acid
Intensity of activity	High intensity
Duration of system	Up to three minutes depending on intensity
Strengths	No delay for oxygen and large fuel stores in the liver, muscles and blood stream Relatively fast fuel breakdown for ATP resynthesis Provides energy for high-intensity activities for up to three minutes Lactic acid can be recycled into fuel for further energy production
Weaknesses	Fatiguing by-product lactic acid reduces pH and enzyme activity Relatively low ATP yield and recovery can be lengthy

Activity

Fill in the blanks in the following paragraph:
The glycolytic energy system serves to provide _____ for ATP resynthesis. Glucose is broken down into pyruvic acid in a series of reactions catalysed by the enzyme _____. This process is known as _____ glycolysis. Due to the lack of oxygen, pyruvic acid is converted into _____ _____ by the enzyme lactate dehydrogenase (LDH), which accumulates, leading to OBLA and early _____.

Aerobic system

The aerobic system kicks in during low- to moderate-intensity activity as the arrival of sufficient oxygen enables continued energy production. The aerobic system utilises around 95 per cent of the potential energy in glucose through three distinct stages:

1 Aerobic glycolysis
2 **Kreb's cycle**
3 **Electron transport chain (ETC).**

Aerobic glycolysis

Aerobic glycolysis in the sarcoplasm converts glucose into pyruvic acid with the enzyme PFK catalysing the reaction. This releases enough energy to resynthesise two moles of ATP. Converting glycogen into glucose (by enzyme GPP) maintains this process for extended periods of time. As oxygen is now in sufficient supply, the pyruvic acid is no longer converted into lactic acid. It goes through a link reaction catalysed by coenzyme A, which produces acetyl CoA. This allows access to the power house of the muscle cell, the **mitochondria.**

Kreb's cycle

Acetyl CoA combines with oxaloacetic acid to form citric acid, which is oxidised through a cycle of reactions. Known as the Kreb's cycle, CO_2, hydrogen and enough energy to resynthesise two moles of ATP are released. This process occurs in the matrix (intracellular fluid) of the mitochondria.

Electron transport chain (ETC)

The hydrogen atoms are carried through the electron transport chain along the cristae (folds of the inner membrane) of the mitochondria by NAD and FAD (hydrogen carriers), splitting into ions (H^+) and electrons (H^-). Hydrogen ions are oxidised and removed as H_2O. Pairs of hydrogen electrons carried by NAD ($NADH_2$) release enough energy to resynthesise 30 moles of ATP and those carried by FAD ($FADH_2$) release enough energy to resynthesise 4 moles of ATP. The overall energy yield of the ETC is 34 moles of ATP.

When all three stages are combined, one mole of glucose yields 38 moles of ATP. This is a highly efficient and most preferable energy system used for long-duration low- to moderate-intensity activities such as marathons, triathlons, cross-country skiing, Tour de France cycling and jogging back onside after a goal has been scored in hockey. The higher the performer's aerobic capacity, the faster oxygen will arrive in plentiful supply and the switch can be made to aerobic energy production.

Key terms

Kreb's cycle: the second stage of the aerobic system producing energy to resynthesise 2 ATP in the mitochondrial matrix.
Electron transport chain (ETC): the third stage of the aerobic system producing energy to resynthesise 34 ATP in the mitochondrial cristae.
Mitochondria: a structure within the cell where aerobic respiration and energy production occur.

Evaluation

To summarise:
- Breakdown of glucose: Glucose + $6O_2$ → $6CO_2$ + $6H_2O$ + energy
- Resynthesis of ATP: Energy + 38P + 38ADP → 38ATP
- Breakdown of ATP: ATP → ADP + P + energy for muscular contraction

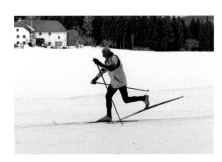

▲ Figure 1.1.6 A highly efficient energy system is required for long-duration, low- to moderate-intensity activities, such as cross-country skiing

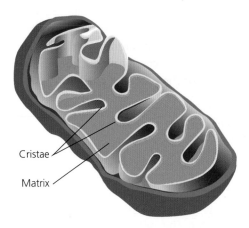

Cristae

Matrix

▲ Figure 1.1.7 The matrix and cristae of the mitochondria

The aerobic system and FFAs

Glycogen stores are large and will fuel the aerobic system for a significant period of time. However, long-distance performers will want to reserve glycogen stores because they can be broken down both aerobically and anaerobically for higher-intensity sections of events or games (such as changes in pace or sprint finishes in a marathon). Triglycerides or fats can also be metabolised aerobically as free fatty acids (FFAs), providing a preferred and huge potential fuel store which conserves glycogen and glucose for those higher-intensity sections.

Upon the release of **lipase**, an enzyme responsible for catalysing the breakdown of fats, triglycerides are converted into FFAs and glycerol. FFAs are converted into acetyl CoA and follow the same path through the Kreb's cycle and electron transport chain as pyruvic acid. FFAs produce more acetyl CoA and a higher energy yield and are therefore preferable for long-distance athletes whose events last more than an hour. However, FFAs require around 15 per cent more oxygen to metabolise and consequently the intensity of activity must remain low.

Key term

Lipase: an enzyme which catalyses the breakdown of triglycerides into free fatty acids (FFAs) and glycerol.

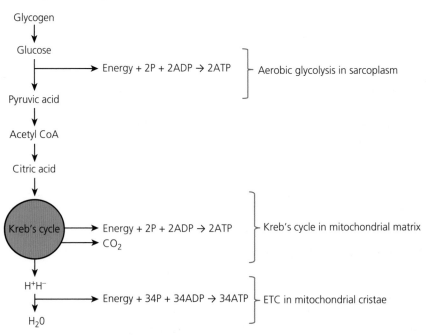

▲ Figure 1.1.8 An overview of the aerobic energy system

To improve the efficiency of the aerobic energy system, aerobic training should be performed. This will improve aerobic capacity, VO_2max, slow oxidative (SO) fibre type recruitment, and mitochondrial size and density. A performer can glycogen load, use pre- and post-event meals and supplement nitrates and caffeine to maximise the body's stores of glycogen and use of triglycerides. Combining the correct training and diet will increase the availability of oxygen, boosting the intensity and duration of performance without the associated effects of fatigue.

▼ Table 1.1.3 The key descriptors, strengths and weaknesses of the aerobic system

Type of reaction	Aerobic (with the presence of oxygen)
Site of reaction	Sarcoplasm, matrix and cristae of mitochondria
Food fuel used	Glycogen/glucose and triglycerides (FFAS)
Controlling enzyme	GPP, PFK, co-enzyme A and lipase
ATP yield	1 mole of glycogen yields up to 38 moles of ATP (1:38)
Specific stages	Aerobic glycolysis, Kreb's cycle and electron transport chain (ETC) Glucose + $6O_2 \rightarrow 6CO_2 + 6H_2O$ + energy (exothermic) Energy + 38P + 38ADP $\rightarrow$ 38ATP (endothermic)
By-products	CO_2 and H_2O
Intensity of activity	Low–moderate/sub-maximal intensity
Duration of system	Three minutes onwards
Strengths	Large fuel stores; triglycerides, FFAs, glycogen and glucose High ATP yield and long duration of energy production No fatiguing by-products
Weaknesses	Delay for oxygen delivery and complex series of reactions Slow energy production limits activity to sub-maximal intensity Triglycerides or FFAs demand around 15 per cent more O_2 for breakdown

ATP resynthesis during exercise of differing intensities and durations

Considering each energy system as separate and responsible totally for resynthesising ATP for a certain activity gives a distorted view of what happens in the muscle cell. At rest we provide almost all energy for ATP resynthesis using the aerobic system; however, when we start to exercise our demand for energy increases significantly and there may not be enough oxygen available to maintain sole aerobic energy production. We must consider how the three energy systems work together depending on the intensity and duration of the activity and the athlete's fitness to provide the overall energy requirement.

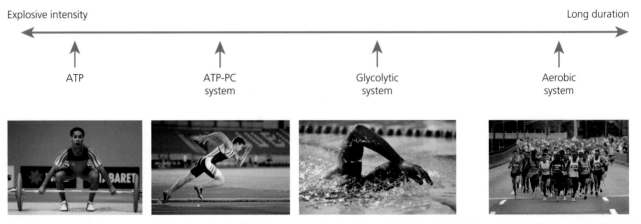

Explosive intensity   Long duration

ATP   ATP-PC system   Glycolytic system   Aerobic system

▲ Figure 1.1.9 The intensity and duration trade-off for energy production

Energy continuum

The **energy continuum** is the relative contribution of each energy system to overall energy production. This will depend on the intensity and duration of the activity. One energy system may be predominant in providing the energy for ATP resynthesis, but in most cases all energy systems will contribute to all activities. For example, in a marathon the majority of the miles will be covered running with the pack at a constant pace; therefore, the aerobic system will be predominant in providing energy for ATP resynthesis. However, when the pace increases, if someone makes a break or an athlete wants to distance themselves from the pack, the glycolytic system will be predominant for this higher-intensity section. Based on the intensity and duration of the activity or sections within the activity, an indication of the contribution each energy system makes to overall energy production can be made. This is important to design effective training and nutritional programmes.

- Intensity very high: duration < 10 seconds
  - In individual activities such as athletic jumps, throws and sprints, where the intensity is very high and duration is 2–10 seconds, the ATP-PC system will be predominant, contributing up to 99 per cent of energy for ATP resynthesis.
- Intensity high: duration 10 seconds to 3 minutes
  - In individual activities such as the 400 m, 200 m freestyle and a competitive squash game, where the intensity is high and duration is between ten seconds and three minutes, the glycolytic system will be predominant, contributing 60–90 per cent of energy for ATP resynthesis.
- Intensity low–moderate: duration >3 minutes
  - In individual activities such as marathons, triathlons and cross-country skiing, where the intensity is moderate but relatively constant for a significant duration, the aerobic system will be predominant, contributing up to 99 per cent of energy for ATP resynthesis.

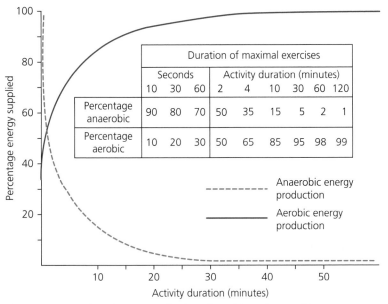

	Duration of maximal exercises								
	Seconds			Activity duration (minutes)					
	10	30	60	2	4	10	30	60	120
Percentage anaerobic	90	80	70	50	35	15	5	2	1
Percentage aerobic	10	20	30	50	65	85	95	98	99

▲ Figure 1.1.10 The relative contribution of aerobic and anaerobic energy production over time

Activity

Summarise the graph shown in Figure 1.1.10 and use a sporting example to explain a specific portion of the data.

Activity

Using a sports paper or magazine, cut out images of different sports or sporting situations and place them on an energy continuum line. Based on intensity and duration, justify which energy system is predominant for energy production.

Intermittent exercise

Intermittent exercise is where the intensity alternates, either during interval training between work and relief intervals or during a game with breaks of play or changes in intensity. For example, a rugby player is required to alternate between various modes of activity such as standing, walking, running, sprinting, tackling and jumping, in comparison with the relatively constant nature of a marathon. Research has shown performing intermittent exercise to be more energy demanding than continuous exercise when the mean running speed is the same, and this places games players in a unique situation, with varying physiological demands as they switch from one energy system's predominance to another.

The point at which an athlete's predominant energy production moves from one energy system to another is known as a **threshold**. A performer can move between any of the energy systems depending on the intensity and duration of the activity and fuels available. For example:

Key terms

Intermittent exercise: activity where the intensity alternates, either during interval training between work and relief intervals or during a game with breaks of play and changes in intensity.
Threshold: the point at which an athlete's predominant energy production moves from one energy system to another.

- ATP-PC/glycolytic threshold: as a wing attack in netball hears the whistle, they will sprint out to receive the centre pass over 3–4 seconds, using ATP predominantly resynthesised by the ATP-PC system.
  However, losing possession leads them to man–man mark for a period of up to one minute to regain possession. The PC stores quickly deplete and the glycolytic system takes over predominant energy production.
- Glycolytic/aerobic threshold: after the counter attack in netball results in a goal being scored, the player jogs back into position ready for the next centre to be taken. The intensity is significantly reduced and there is sufficient oxygen available for the aerobic system to take over to provide most of the energy for ATP resynthesis.

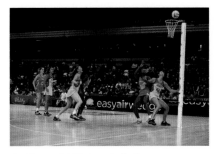

▲ Figure 1.1.11 A netball player can move between different energy systems depending on the intensity of the game

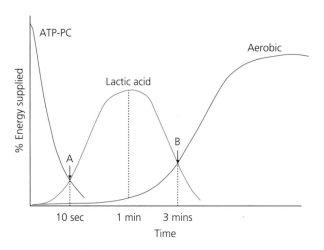

A = ATP-PC LA threshold
The point at which ATP-PC energy system is exhausted and lactic acid system prevails

B = LA O$_2$ threshold
The point at which lactic acid system is exhausted and the aerobic system takes over

▲ Figure 1.1.12 The percentage of energy supplied by each energy system over time

Recovery periods

Predominantly anaerobic activities such as basketball and netball rely heavily on the ATP-PC and glycolytic systems. Although PC stores quickly deplete in around eight seconds, they are also quickly replenished – 50 per cent in just 30 seconds and 100 per cent after 3 minutes – making timeouts an essential tactical part of play. Equally, oxygen stored in the **myoglobin** depleted after bouts of exhaustive exercise can be fully relinked within three minutes of rest or low-intensity exercise. The quarter- and half-time breaks aid recovery and maintain the intensity of the game for both performers and spectators.

Blood lactate levels can rise dramatically with prolonged high-intensity bouts such as an exhaustive tennis rally, and also slowly accumulate with repeated use of the glycolytic system without sufficient relief, in 400 m training, for example. With the correct **work to relief ratios** and sufficient oxygen supply, lactic acid can be broken down and removed. Lactic acid removal is aided by low-intensity activity, which maintains blood flow and oxygen transport. Therefore, during intermittent exercise, lactic acid levels can fluctuate, building up and initiating fatigue during high-intensity bouts, then partially cleared during relief intervals to prolong the duration of activity.

Key terms

Myoglobin: a red protein in the muscle cell responsible for carrying and storing oxygen.
Work to relief ratio: the volume of relief in relation to the volume of work performed.

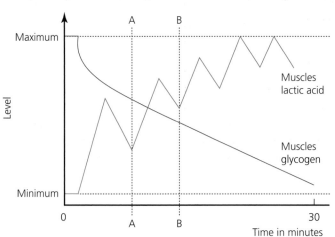

▲ Figure 1.1.13 Lactic acid and glycogen response to a 30-minute interval training session

Activity

Summarise the graph in Figure 1.1.13. Considering the nature of lactic acid levels, describe the type of activity most likely being performed and consider the relationship between muscle glycogen and lactic acid between points A and B.

Recovery periods also present opportunities for rehydration and glycogen/ glucose replenishment for athletes competing for longer than 60 minutes. Tennis players, team game players, triathletes and Tour de France cyclists are just some of the many athletes who use glucose tablets, gels, bananas and isotonic drinks in breaks of play, changeovers and lower-intensity intervals to maintain glycogen stores and replace lost glucose.

RESEARCH IN FOCUS

Fernandez *et al.* (*British Journal of Sports Medicine*, 2006) compiled a review on the intensity of tennis match play. They found tennis to be characterised by intermittent exercise, short 4–10 s, high-intensity bouts, interrupted by longer duration 60–90 s bouts with underlying periods of moderate- to low-intensity activity. Recovery periods controlled by ITF (International Tennis Federation) rules are limited to 20 s between points, 90 s between changeovers and 120 s between sets, giving a mean work:relief ratio of between 1:1 and 1:4.

Modification to the scoring system, match duration, playing surface and ball type all affect the physiological demands of tennis matches lasting from one to more than five hours. During long, intense rallies, blood lactate levels can reach 8 mmol/l, although frequent relief intervals are probably sufficient to metabolise lactate effectively and in general lactate levels remain low (1.8–2.8 mmol/l).

Evidence suggested all three energy systems are required during match play, requiring specific training for ATP-PC, glycolytic and aerobic efficiency. Interval training replicating distances and activities related to competition are preferable.

Fitness level

An athlete with a high aerobic capacity or **VO$_2$max** has an efficient cardiovascular and respiratory system to inspire, transport and utilise great volumes of oxygen. This increases the intensity at which they can perform as a percentage of their VO$_2$max before OBLA is reached and fatigue sets in. Buffering capacity is increased, limiting the effects of lactic acid accumulation, and the removal of lactic acid is improved as the muscles are flushed with oxygenated blood flow. Sufficient oxygen will also arrive onsite earlier than in untrained performers, minimising time spent in the glycolytic system accumulating lactic acid. Another advantage of a high aerobic capacity is the use of FFAs (the most energy-rich fuel), which demand 15 per cent more oxygen to break down. In trained performers, the additional oxygen demand to use FFAs can be met, which conserves glycogen stores for higher-intensity bouts of activity, increasing the duration of performance.

Key term

VO$_2$max: maximum volume of oxygen inspired, transported and utilised per minute during exhaustive exercise.

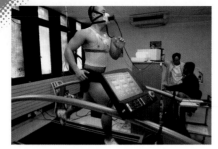

▲ Figure 1.1.14 An athlete performing a VO$_2$ max test

IN THE NEWS

Mo Farah has the 'triple-double', a third consecutive global championship double triumph in the 5,000 m and 10,000 m events: London, Moscow and Beijing. With the constant change and increase in pace leading to sprint finishes, Mo Farah will suffer micro-damage to the muscle fibres, tissue inflammation and a severe accumulation of lactic acid after the first event. After just a few days he must be prepared to face world-class fresh competitors in the second race. These events combine anaerobic and aerobic fitness and Mo Farah will train to delay OBLA to keep lactic acid levels near baseline until exhaustive exercise. He will use cooling aids, massage and nutritional support to be performance ready.

Additional factors will affect the relative contribution of the energy systems to overall energy production, such as the following for a games player:

● Position of the player: for example, a goalkeeper's aerobic energy system may be predominant, with a small percentage from the ATP-PC system for very high-intensity dives, kicks and defensive play, whereas a central midfielder's aerobic system will be required to jog back into position and track play, their glycolytic system will be used for counter attacks and set pieces, and the ATP-PC system for high-intensity sprints into the box, shots on goal or tackles.

● Tactics and strategies used: for example, man–man marking will raise the intensity compared with zonal marking and will require a larger contribution from the anaerobic energy systems.

● Level of competition: in a hard match with tough competition, the intensity will be far higher, increasing the contribution from the anaerobic energy systems and relying more heavily on defensive players. In a relatively easy match with weak competition, the intensity will be lower, increasing the contribution of the aerobic energy system.

● Structure of the game: field games such as rugby, football and hockey are played on a large pitch, increasing the duration and lowering the intensity of runs and set plays. This increases the contribution of the aerobic energy system. Court games such as basketball and netball are played on small courts, increasing the intensity and decreasing the duration of runs and set plays. This increases the contribution of the anaerobic energy systems.

Activity

For a game player of your choice, draw a bar chart showing the percentage of energy supplied by each energy system. Justify your answer with specific examples.

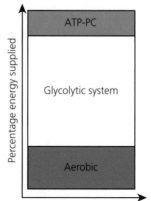

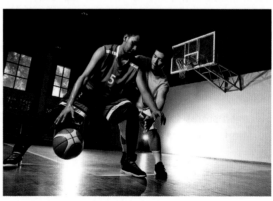

▲ Figure 1.1.15 The relative contribution of each energy system to overall energy production of a basketball player

Summary

Energy for exercise centres on ATP, its role and resynthesis via the three main energy systems and how these energy systems interact during differing intensities and durations of activity.

- ATP is a high-energy compound broken down by ATPase to provide an immediate source of energy for muscular contraction exothermically. ATP provides energy for explosive activities, depletes after 2–3 seconds and can be resynthesised to maintain energy production using energy from food fuel breakdown.
- The ATP-PC energy system resynthesises ATP from the breakdown of phosphocreatine (PC) by creatine kinase in a coupled reaction.
  - PC $\rightarrow$ C + P + energy in an anaerobic reaction in the sarcoplasm yielding one mole of ATP, for very high-intensity activities lasting 2–10 seconds.
- The glycolytic energy system resynthesises ATP from the breakdown of glycogen by GPP and glucose by PFK.
  - Glucose $\rightarrow$ pyruvic acid + energy in the sarcoplasm yielding two moles of ATP, for high-intensity activities lasting ten seconds to three minutes.
  - Pyruvic acid $\rightarrow$ lactic acid by LDH due to anaerobic conditions which accumulates to reach OBLA, causing fatigue.
- The aerobic energy system resynthesises ATP from the breakdown of glycogen, glucose and FFAs by GPP, PFK or lipase.
  - Aerobic glycolysis: glucose $\rightarrow$ pyruvic acid + energy by PFK in the sarcoplasm. Kreb's cycle: acetyl CoA $\rightarrow$ CO_2 + H + energy in the matrix of the mitochondria. Electron transport chain where H $\rightarrow$ H_2O + energy in the cristae of the mitochondria, yielding 38 moles of ATP for low- to moderate-intensity activities lasting more than three minutes.
- The energy continuum is the relative contribution of each energy system to overall energy production depending on intensity and duration. Each energy system can be expressed; for example, a central midfielder's energy demand may be supplied 60 per cent by the aerobic system, 30 per cent by the glycolytic system and 10 per cent by the ATP-PC system.
  - The energy continuum will also depend on the performer's fitness, recovery intervals, type of activity, tactics employed and player position.

1 Answer the following statements as true or false:
   a ATP is the only immediately available source of energy for muscular contraction.
   b Phosphocreatine is broken down, releasing energy for muscular contraction.
   c The energy yield of the ATP-PC system is two moles of ATP.
   d The glycolytic system's main disadvantage is the production of lactic acid, which causes muscular fatigue.
   e The breakdown of glucose through the process of glycolysis can be both anaerobic and aerobic.
   f The Kreb's cycle reactions occur in the cristae of the mitochondria.
   g The electron transport chain produces large quantities of energy for ATP resynthesis.
   h The energy continuum is the relative contribution of each energy system to overall energy production and depends on the intensity and duration of an activity.

2 Identify the key terms from the following statements:
   a When the products of one reaction are used in another reaction.
   b The enzyme responsible for ATP breakdown.
   c The end product of glycolysis.
   d The point at which blood lactate levels reach 4 mmol/l.
   e The point where one energy system takes over predominant energy production from another.

Practice questions

1 Explain the role of ATP in muscular contraction.   (4 marks)

2 Describe the effects of insufficient oxygen supply on the breakdown of glucose for ATP resynthesis.   (5 marks)

3 Define the energy continuum and using a team game of your choice, justify when and why all three energy systems are used.   (6 marks)

4 Using the ATP-PC energy system as an example, describe what is meant by the term 'coupled reaction'. Describe how the structural and functional characteristics of fast glycolytic (FG) muscle fibre types enhance the efficiency of the ATP-PC energy system.   (20 marks)

1.2 Recovery, altitude and heat

Understanding the specification

By the end of this chapter you should be able to demonstrate knowledge and understanding of the key role recovery plays in returning the body to its pre-exercise state and how different environmental conditions affect performance.

The recovery process:

- excess post-exercise oxygen consumption (EPOC)
- fast components of EPOC
- slow components of EPOC
- training and performance implications of recovery.

Environmental effects:

- the effect of altitude on the cardiovascular and respiratory systems
- acclimatisation and timing of arrival for performance at altitude
- the effect of heat on the cardiovascular and respiratory systems
- temperature regulation and the cardiovascular drift.

The recovery process

Athletes have the potential to motivate, inspire, entertain and make the viewing public hold their breath in anticipation of broken records and personal bests. However, with packed event calendars that see athletes travel all over the world and compete in back-to-back events, there is nothing more disappointing than watching an athlete underperform. In this day and age recovery is hugely important to maintain the intensity of both training and competition.

Excess post-exercise oxygen consumption

By the time the exercise or performance ends, the athlete's body is in a state of fatigue. Myoglobin has lost its stores of oxygen, ATP, PC and glycogen stores may be depleted, and lactic acid levels may be high, potentially leading to feelings of exhaustion. Post exercise the body enters a period of recovery, with the primary aim of returning the body to a pre-exercise state where all stored fuels are complete and the blood and muscle tissue are free of by-products.

To return the body to a pre-exercise state, energy is required. Continued aerobic energy production fulfils this additional energy requirement and is termed **excess post-exercise oxygen consumption (EPOC)**. EPOC is also known as oxygen debt and represents the volume of oxygen required post exercise to return the body to a pre-exercise state.

Oxygen consumption can be plotted against time to show the **oxygen deficit** (the volume of oxygen required to complete an activity entirely aerobically): oxygen consumption during exercise and EPOC. The graph in Figure 1.2.1 clearly shows oxygen consumption post exercise decreases rapidly before gradually returning to resting levels. This represents the two distinct stages of EPOC:

1 The fast component of recovery.

2 The slow component of recovery.

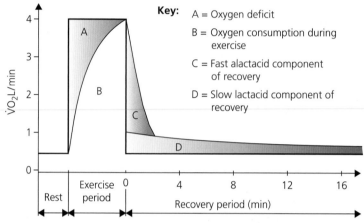

▲ Figure 1.2.1 Oxygen consumption during exercise and recovery

EPOC is always present, regardless of the intensity of exercise. However, the size of the oxygen deficit and EPOC may differ depending on activity intensity and duration. During low-intensity aerobic activities there is a small oxygen deficit as steady-state oxygen consumption is quickly met, limiting the use of the anaerobic energy systems and lactic acid accumulation. In contrast, during high-intensity anaerobic activities there is a large oxygen deficit as oxygen supply does not meet demand and lactic acid accumulates, readily reaching OBLA quickly. EPOC needs to be large enough to counteract the oxygen deficit and provide oxygen to resaturate myoglobin and satisfy additional energy requirements.

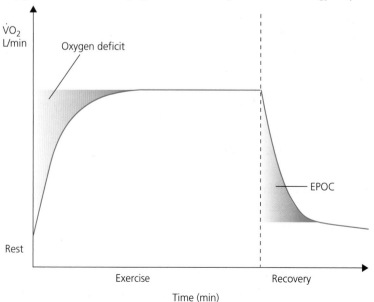

▲ Figure 1.2.2 Oxygen consumption during low-intensity activity

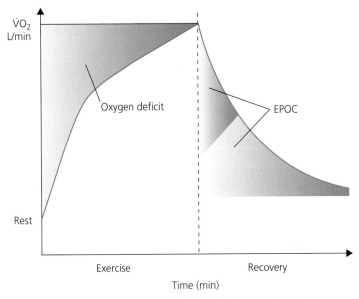

▲ Figure 1.2.3 Oxygen consumption during high-intensity activity

Fast alactacid component of recovery

As a performer enters recovery, the first stage is known as the **fast alactacid** (before lactic acid) component and accounts for around 10 per cent of EPOC. This component shows the volume of oxygen (approximately 1–4 litres) required to complete the initial jobs to return the body to a pre-exercise state, including the:

- replenishment of blood and muscle oxygen
- resynthesis of ATP and PC stores.

Replenishment of blood and muscle oxygen

During exercise oxygen is dissociated from haemoglobin in the blood stream and myoglobin in the muscle cells to fuel aerobic glycolysis and aerobic energy production. Within the first minute of EPOC, oxygen resaturates the blood stream, associating with haemoglobin, and within three minutes restoring the oxy–myoglobin link in the muscle cells.

Resynthesis of ATP and PC stores

During exercise muscle cells' stores of ATP and PC are depleted to fuel the ATP-PC energy system. Within the first three minutes of EPOC, aerobic energy production continues, providing the energy to resynthesise ATP and PC. Essential for this resynthesis is the restoration of muscle phosphagen (P), providing the phosphate required to restore the high-energy bonds to ADP and creatine. Restoration of muscle phosphagen takes approximately 30 seconds for 50 per cent and 3 minutes for full restoration. With energy and phosphates, ATP and PC resynthesis can occur. This can be summarised as:

- Energy + P + ADP $\rightarrow$ ATP
- Energy + P + C $\rightarrow$ PC

Slow lactacid component of recovery

After the fast alactacid component of recovery the body enters the slow lactacid component. This portion of EPOC shows the volume of oxygen

Key term

Fast alactacid recovery: the initial fast stage of EPOC where oxygen consumed within three minutes resaturates haemoglobin and myoglobin stores and provides the energy for ATP and PC resynthesis.

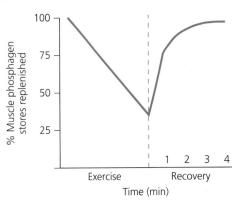

▲ Figure 1.2.4 Muscle phosphagen restoration post exercise

(approximately 5–8 litres) required to complete the more complex and time-consuming jobs to return the body to a pre-exercise state. These include the:

- provision of energy to maintain ventilation, circulation and body temperature
- removal of lactic acid and replenishment of glycogen.

Ventilation and circulation

During exercise respiratory rate and depth and heart rate rise significantly to provide the muscle cells with the necessary quantities of oxygen for energy production. Post exercise these remain elevated, then decrease gradually to resting levels to maximise the delivery of oxygen and the removal of by-products such as carbon dioxide in the plasma, as carbonic acid (H_2CO_3) and carbaminohaemoglobin ($HbCO_2$). Although this provides the necessary removal of carbon dioxide and intake and transportation of oxygen to continue aerobic energy production, there is an energy cost attached which accounts for around 1–2 per cent of EPOC.

Body temperature

During exercise it is common for heat production to exceed heat removal, causing a rise in core body temperature. For every 1° Celsius rise in body temperature the metabolic rate increases by around 13–15 per cent. Post exercise the elevated temperature remains, potentially for several hours after vigorous exercise, accounting for as much as 60–70 per cent of the slow lactacid component of EPOC.

Removal of lactic acid and replenishment of glycogen

During anaerobic exercise or activity with high-intensity bouts lactic acid will accumulate within the muscles and capillary beds, causing local muscular fatigue as an athlete hits OBLA. Post exercise lactic acid readily converts back to pyruvic acid and is then either oxidised or converted into glycogen:

1 Approximately 50–75 per cent of pyruvic acid is oxidised in the mitochondria, re-entering the Kreb's cycle and electron transport chain to produce CO_2, H_2O and energy aerobically (review your knowledge in Chapter 1.1).

2 Approximately 10–25 per cent of pyruvic acid is reconverted into glucose to top up blood supplies and glycogen to be stored in the muscles and liver, through processes called **gluconeogenesis** and **glyconeogenesis**.

3 Small amounts of pyruvic acid are also converted into protein by the Cori cycle in the liver and removed from the body in the sweat and urine.

The removal of lactic acid also relies on the buffering capacity of the blood, which neutralises its effects. Hydrogen carbonate ions produced by the kidneys absorb hydrogen ions released by lactic acid and form carbonic acid (H_2CO_3). Carbonic acid can be broken down to form carbon dioxide and H_2O for removal at the lungs.

Lactic acid removal takes on average around one hour; however, it can take up to 24 hours depending on the intensity of exercise, volumes of lactic acid accumulated and recovery methods used. This has major implications for lactate performers' training and nutritional regimes.

Key term

Gluconeogenesis/ glyconeogenesis: the formation of glucose/glycogen from substrates such as pyruvic acid.

Study hint

Lactic acid should not be described as a waste product as it can be readily converted back into pyruvic acid and used as a fuel. It can be described as a harmful by-product of the glycolytic system.

Fill in the blanks in the following paragraph:

The fast _____ component of EPOC requires 1–4 litres of _____ to complete the first part of the recovery process. Oxygen resaturates _____ in the blood stream and _____ in the muscle cells. Oxygen also continues aerobic energy production, providing the energy and phosphates required to resynthesise _____ and _____ stores. For full restoration _____ minutes are required; however, 50 per cent restoration can be completed in just 30 seconds.

During exercise, hormone levels also rise. Hormones such as epinephrine, norepinephrine and cortisol aid fuel mobilisation, neural transmission and muscle contraction. Until these hormones are cleared from the blood stream they require energy and therefore oxygen, which account for a significant part of EPOC.

Implications of recovery on training

Knowledge and understanding of EPOC and the recovery processes are essential for both athlete and coach to maintain training efficiency and ensure repeated peak performances. At an elite level each athlete's recovery is individually designed following general principles based on the use of a warm up, active recovery, cooling aids, intensity planning, work:relief ratios and the correct nutrition.

1   Warm up. By performing a warm up, respiratory, heart and metabolic rates increase, accelerating use of the aerobic system, which minimises the time spent using the anaerobic energy systems for energy production and the associated lactic acid accumulation. This will reduce the oxygen deficit, limiting the amount of oxygen required to 'pay it back' during EPOC.

2   Active recovery. Using an active cool down maintains respiratory and heart rates, flushing the muscle and capillary beds with oxygenated blood flow. This speeds up the removal of lactic acid and reduces the length of the slow lactacid component of EPOC, essential if there are repeated bouts of exercise on the same day. A moderate-intensity, active recovery 40–60 per cent VO$_2$max is advisable for athletes who accumulate lactic acid during their performance; however, it may have little benefit for aerobic athletes who achieve a steady-state oxygen consumption. A passive recovery may help reduce the temperature and metabolic rate, diminishing the energy cost on EPOC.

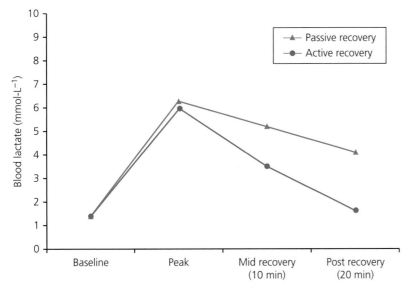

▲ Figure 1.2.5 Effect of mode of recovery on blood lactate levels

3   Cooling aids. Aids, such as ice baths, can be used post event to lower the muscle and blood temperature to resting levels, reducing the metabolic rate and demand on the slow lactacid component of EPOC. Cooling aids can also be used after an event to speed up lactic acid removal, reduce muscle damage and decrease delayed onset muscle soreness (DOMS).

4   Intensity of training. The intensity of training should be monitored using heart rate to ensure training intensity is specific to the energy system and muscle fibre type, and mirrors the demands of the activity, overloading to progressively create an appropriate adaptation:

    a   High-intensity training will increase muscle mass, ATP and PC storage capacity, boosting the efficiency of the fast component of recovery.

    b   High-intensity training will increase the tolerance to lactic acid, increase buffering capacity and delay OBLA, reducing the demand in the slow lactacid component of EPOC.

    c   Low–moderate intensity training will increase aerobic capacity, and respiratory and cardiovascular efficiency. An earlier move to aerobic energy production minimises lactic acid build-up, delaying OBLA, and maximises oxygen delivery post exercise during EPOC.

5   Work:relief ratios. Based on the predominant energy system required in a physical activity, training intensity and the correct work:relief ratio can maximise recovery:

    a   For speed and explosive strength-based performers predominantly using the ATP-PC system, such as a 100 m sprinter, a work:relief ratio of 1:3+ should give sufficient time for ATP and PC stores to resynthesise within the session.

    b   For lactate tolerance and high-intensity muscular endurance performers predominantly using the glycolytic system, such as an 800 m runner, a work:relief ratio of 1:2 should give sufficient recovery to continue training but encourage lactic acid accumulation to increase tolerance and buffering capacity.

    c   For aerobic capacity or endurance performers predominantly using the aerobic system, such as a triathlete, a work:relief ratio of 1:1 or 1:0.5 will promote adaptation, and delay OBLA and muscular fatigue.

6   Strategies and tactics. A coach should use timeouts and substitutions to allow 30-second relief intervals for 50 per cent ATP and PC replenishment. Performers can delay play, for example, by a team maintaining possession in defence or a tennis player changing rackets, lowering the intensity to allow relief intervals to clear lactic acid and resynthesise ATP and PC stores. Set plays and marking or running strategies can also lower the intensity, delaying OBLA and fatigue.

7   Nutrition. The correct pre-, during- and post-event nutrition can help the performer to maximise fuel stores, delay fatigue, reduce lactic acid accumulation and speed up recovery:

    a   To maximise PC stores a performer may load creatine, phosphagen and protein, increasing the efficiency of the ATP-PC system and the fast stage of recovery.

    b   To maximise glucose and glycogen a performer may carbohydrate load, and use pre-event, during-event and post-event meals and snacks, maximising the efficiency of the glycolytic and aerobic systems and the slow stage of recovery.

c To tolerate the effects of lactic acid a performer may use bicarbonate to enhance the buffering process. Those training close to the lactate threshold may use nitrates to reduce the oxygen cost of exercise and speed up recovery times with enhanced oxygenated blood flow.

▼ Table 1.2.1 An overview of the implications of EPOC and the recovery process on training aims

Training aim	Predominant energy system	Recovery strategies
Speed/explosive strength	ATP-PC	Warm up Work:relief ratio of 1:3+ with full three-minute recovery between sets Timeouts and substitutions Creatine supplementation and phosphate loading
Lactate tolerance	Glycolytic	Warm up Active recovery Cooling aids Work:relief ratio of 1:2 Timeouts, substitutions, delaying play, set pieces and marking/running strategies Pre-event, during-event, post-event carbohydrate meal/snack Bicarbonate (soda loading) and nitrate supplementation
Aerobic capacity	Aerobic	Warm up Passive recovery Cooling aids Work:relief ratio of 1:1–1:0.5 Delaying play, set pieces and marking/running strategies Carbohydrate loading, pre-event, during-event and post-event meal/snack Nitrate supplementation

Environmental effects on the body systems

Athletes who compete in the open air must face a huge range of conditions during their competitive year. Elite footballers who are used to competing at sea level in mild, often wet conditions in the UK must also maximise performance at **altitude** and in extremes of heat. The 2010 South Africa World Cup included six venues over 1,200 m above sea level and two around 1,750 m in Johannesburg. 2014 saw Estadio Nacional in Brasilia standing at 1,172 m above sea level, 30°C and 80 per cent **humidity** in Manaus, and up to 37°C and 70 per cent humidity in Cuiaba. The World Cup awarded to Qatar in 2022 has faced fierce criticism over the soaring desert heat, which regularly tops 50°C, and consequently FIFA has moved the competition to a November and December schedule. This move will disrupt top leagues in Europe and displace Africa's continental championship.

Differing environmental conditions affect the efficiency of the cardiovascular and respiratory systems and can dramatically affect performance and even health of both athletes and spectators. Athletes and coaches must prepare for these conditions and alter strategies to ensure peak performances can be maintained.

Activity

A football player has some physiological measurements taken three minutes into recovery after the match has finished. PC stores, heart rate and respiratory rate are high, blood lactate levels are moderately high and glycogen stores are low. Consider these levels, the physiological processes that have occurred leading to these levels, and the physiological processes still required to return the body to a pre-exercise state. Write a maximum of 800 words in an extended answer format.

Activity

Based on the intensity, duration and demands of your preferred sport, what key pieces of knowledge should you incorporate into your recovery routine?

Key terms

Altitude: the height or elevation of an area above sea level.
Humidity: the amount of water vapour in the atmospheric air.

Key terms

Barometric pressure: the pressure exerted by the earth's atmosphere at any given point.
Partial pressure: the pressure exerted by an individual gas held in a mixture of gases.

Effect of altitude on the cardiovascular and respiratory systems

Altitude is the height of an area above sea level. As altitude increases, **barometric pressure** decreases. Even though the composition of the air remains the same with 20.9 per cent of oxygen, the **partial pressure** of oxygen (pO_2) decreases, which has a severe impact on performance.

▼ Table 1.2.2 The decrease in pO_2 with an increase in altitude

Altitude (m)	Sporting activity	Barometric pressure (mmHg)	pO_2 (mmHg)
Sea level	Marathon: London	760	159
1,319	Winter Olympics: Salt Lake City	654	137
3,600	Football: Hernando Siles Stadium, La Paz	499	105
8,848	Mountaineering: summit Mount Everest	253	43

All gases move down a pressure gradient from an area of high to low partial pressure, diffusing from the alveolar air to the capillary blood and then to the muscle cells. The greater the **diffusion** gradient, the faster the oxygen will move from one area to another. At rest the pO_2 in the deoxygenated capillary blood arriving back at the alveoli is around 40 mmHg. The greater the altitude, the greater the negative impact on the diffusion gradient:

- At sea level pO_2 is 159 mmHg, giving a diffusion gradient of 119 to the capillary blood.
- At 3,600 m above sea level pO_2 is 105 mmHg, giving a diffusion gradient of 65 (45 per cent reduction) to the capillary blood.
- At 8,800 m above sea level on the summit of Everest pO_2 is around 43 mmHg, giving a diffusion gradient of just 3. This severely hampers oxygen **diffusion** into the blood stream, forcing most mountaineers to turn to supplementary oxygen.

Key term

Diffusion: the movement of a gas across a membrane down a gradient from an area of high pressure (or concentration) to an area of low pressure (or concentration).

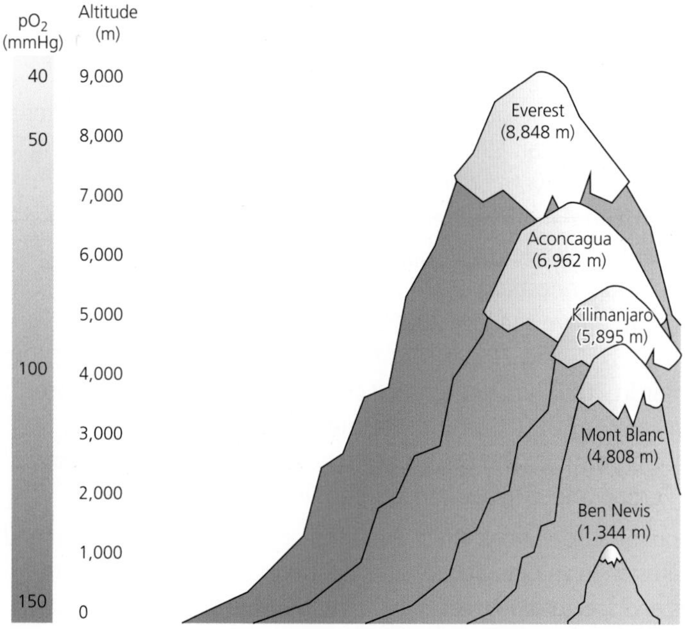

▲ Figure 1.2.6 The relationship between altitude and partial pressure of oxygen

If an athlete competes at high altitude, the rate of oxygen diffusion decreases, reducing haemoglobin saturation, which results in poor transport of oxygen to the muscle tissues for aerobic energy production. As a result:

- breathing frequency increases both at rest and during exercise in an attempt to maintain oxygen consumption
- blood volume decreases as within the first few hours of altitude exposure plasma volume decreases by up to 25 per cent to increase the density of red blood cells in an attempt to maximise oxygen transportation
- stroke volume decreases within the first few hours at altitude during sub-maximal exercise, which increases heart rate to maintain and slightly raise cardiac output
- maximal cardiac output, stroke volume and heart rate decrease with altitude during maximum-intensity exercise.

This combines to reduce aerobic capacity and VO$_2$max, impacting on both the intensity and duration for which an athlete can perform. Results show altitude has little effect on performance below 1,500 m; however, above this height the respiratory and cardiovascular systems become increasingly hampered and for every 1,000 m above 1,500 m altitude VO$_2$max drops by around 8–11 per cent. At the summit of Everest an average sea level VO$_2$max of 62 ml/kg/min can drop to just 15 ml/kg/min. This places greater demand on the anaerobic energy systems to maintain energy production, leading to increased lactic acid production at any sub-maximal intensity and early fatigue.

Coaches must prepare the athletes for performance at altitude and allow extra time and practice, increase work:relief ratios, consider more frequent substitutions and supplement oxygen on the sidelines, for example, in ice hockey or between heats in skating and skiing, to aid recovery.

Extend your knowledge

Anaerobic events lasting less than one minute, such as sprinting, throwing and jumping activities, are unaffected at moderate altitudes. However, higher altitudes have a lower air density (around a 3 per cent reduction every 305 m), which decreases aerodynamic drag and air resistance, resulting in faster speeds in winter sports such as alpine skiing and speed skating. Winter Olympics set at altitude, such as the 2002 Salt Lake City Games, see higher volumes of records broken than lower-altitude games. High altitudes can also affect timing and technical components in skill sports as feedback from balance and proprioception (perception of movement and orientation) will differ and projectiles will move through the air differently. For example, ski jumpers are required to change the angle of their lean depending on altitude of performance.

Activity

Using an example, choose two performers, one who relies on the glycolytic system and one who relies on the aerobic system. Compare gaseous exchange and performance at sea level to high altitude.

Study hint

Recap your anatomy and physiology knowledge of the cardiovascular and respiratory systems from Book 1, chapter 1.2.

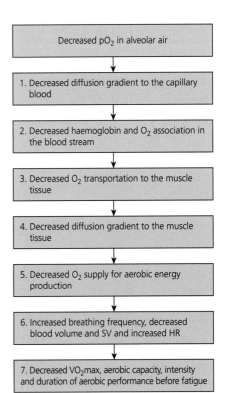

▲ Figure 1.2.7 Overview of the acute effects of high altitude on the cardiovascular and respiratory systems

Acclimatisation

Acclimatisation is a process where an athlete gradually adapts to a change in their environment, in this sense the lower pO_2 in the atmospheric air at altitude. No matter how long an individual spends at altitude prior to the event, they will never fully compensate and regain their sea-level VO_2max. However, for endurance athletes who are reliant on oxygen for aerobic energy production, acclimatisation is essential prior to performance to minimise the impact of the decreased pO_2. Altitude starts to have an effect around 1,500 m and although different people acclimatise at different speeds, guidelines allow:

- 3–5 days for low-altitude performance (1,000–2,000 m)
- 1–2 weeks for moderate-altitude performance (2,000–3,000 m)
- 2+ weeks for high altitude (3,000 m+) whereby athletes going above 3,000 m should sleep no more than 300 m higher each day and have regular rest days to prevent altitude sickness
- 4+ weeks for extreme altitude (5,000–5,500 m); for example, climbers will spend at least one month at base camp before making a summit attempt on Everest.

Extend your knowledge

Estadio Hernando Siles in La Paz, Bolivia is one of the highest stadiums in the world, standing around 3,600 m above sea level. Visiting football teams regularly protest, saying the altitude gives the home side an unfair advantage, especially the double World Cup-winning side Argentina, which didn't record a victory at Estadio Hernando Siles from 1973 to 2005. A shake-up in international football legislation in 2007 led to FIFA declaring no qualifying match could be played over 2,500 m above sea level; however, an outcry led to the following acclimatisation criteria:

- above 2,500 m: three days' acclimatisation recommended
- above 2,750 m: seven days' acclimatisation recommended
- above 3,000 m: games not generally permitted without a minimum two-week acclimatisation.

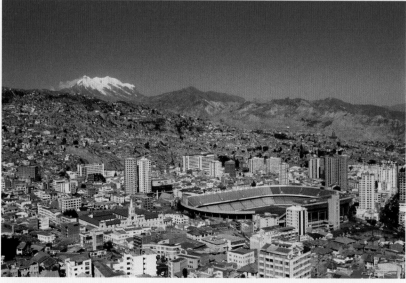

▲ Figure 1.2.8 The Hernando Siles Stadium in La Paz, Bolivia (3,600 m above sea level)

The important benefits of acclimatisation for the cardiovascular and respiratory systems are as follows:

- Release of **erythropoietin** increases within three hours of altitude exposure, peaking 24–48 hours later, which increases red blood cell production. With six weeks' exposure to 4,540 m altitude, the concentration of red blood cells can increase by 14 per cent.
- Breathing rate and ventilation stabilise, however remain elevated at rest and during exercise when compared with sea level.
- Stroke volume and cardiac output reduce as oxygen extraction becomes more efficient. After ten days' acclimatisation, cardiac output is lower at any sub-maximal intensity when compared with sea level while heart rate remains elevated.
- There is reduced incidence of altitude sickness, headaches, breathlessness, poor sleep and lack of appetite.

Exercise in the heat

Exercising in the heat can severely affect performance, disrupt scheduling and have serious consequences for the health of an athlete or spectator. FIFA decided to move the Qatar World Cup in 2022 away from the summer 50°C desert heat on health and safety grounds to the winter months, with the final to be played on 18 December. This was despite the organising committee's promises of revolutionary cooling technologies for stadiums, training areas and fan zones.

IN THE NEWS

Athletes will risk the hottest weather in more than a century at the 2020 Tokyo Olympic Games, highlighting concern over global sporting events in extreme conditions. 2015 saw summer temperatures soar to 38°C and the high humidity in Tokyo, average 71 per cent, will make it feel even hotter – up to 63°C. Under these conditions the men's marathon would be the hottest in at least 120 years, since Paris in 1900 where over half of the entrants withdrew due to exhaustion as temperatures hit an estimated 35–39°C. The events that pose the biggest risk are the marathon and the 10,000 m due to the duration of the races and accumulation of heat within the body.

Normal human body temperature is 37°C, with a daily rise and fall of no more than 1°C. **Thermoregulation** is the process that allows the body to maintain its internal core temperature, which is essential for an individual's health. **Thermoreceptors** deep in the core of the body sense a change in temperature. If core temperature rises, metabolic heat is transported by the circulating blood to the surface of the body and released largely by convection and evaporation (sweat). Sweating has a cooling effect on the body, removing excess heat quickly. Sweating, although critical for heat loss, leads to fluid loss. An athlete exercising in the heat can lose around 2–3 litres per hour, which if not replaced decreases blood volume and causes **dehydration**. Dehydration will impair the body's ability to thermoregulate and core temperature will rise. The rate of heat loss through sweating is affected by humidity (the amount of water in the atmospheric air); low

Key term

Hyperthermia: significantly raised core body temperature.

Study hint

Do not confuse hyperthermia, significantly high core body temperature, with hypothermia, which is the opposite, significantly low core body temperature.

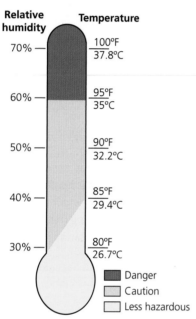

▲ Figure 1.2.9 The heat equation. High humidity + high temperature + physical work = danger

Key term

Cardiovascular drift: upward drift in heart rate during sustained steady-state activity associated with an increase in body temperature.

humidity increases sweating, whereas high humidity decreases sweating and the cooling process.

A rise in core body temperature of several degrees can affect physical performance and, if unlimited, an athlete can enter **hyperthermia**. The three most important causes of increased core body temperature in athletes are:

1 High and prolonged exercise intensities.

2 High air temperatures.

3 High relative humidity.

Hyperthermia is common if an athlete pushes themselves too fast, for too long in too hot and humid conditions.

During prolonged exercise in the heat, the increased rate of muscular contraction and chemical reactions produce metabolic heat, which may not be removed from the body quickly enough to maintain core body temperature. This can cause **cardiovascular drift**: an upward drift in heart rate associated with a rise in body temperature (1°C increases heart rate by 10 bpm). For the exercising athlete the redirection of blood flow to the skin for cooling limits blood flow to the muscles and venous return and the rising core temperature alters the function of protein molecules, such as enzymes and receptors, and affects the rate of chemical reactions.

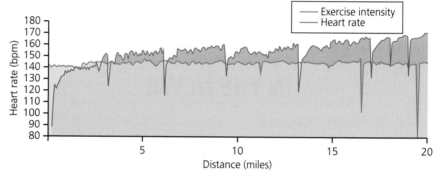

▲ Figure 1.2.10 Cardiovascular drift. The upward drift in heart rate during steady state prolonged exercise

The effect of heat, humidity and the body's thermoregulatory response on the cardiovascular system:

● Dilation of arterioles and capillaries to the skin, leading to:
  ● increased blood flow and blood pooling in the limbs.
● Decreased blood volume, venous return, stroke volume, cardiac output and blood pressure, leading to:
  ● increased heart rate to compensate
  ● increased strain on the cardiovascular system
  ● reduced oxygen transport to the working muscles.

▼ Table 1.2.3 The rate of metabolic heat production from various body compartments at rest and during strenuous exercise

	Heat production		
	Body mass (%)	Rest	Exercise
Brain	2	16	1
Trunk	34	56	8
Muscle and skin	56	18	90
Other	8	10	1

Source: Modified from Wenger, C.B. and Hardy, J.D. (1990) 'Temperature regulation and exposure to heat and cold', in Lehmann, J.F. (ed.) *Therapeutic Heat and Cold*, Baltimore, MD: Williams & Wilkins, pp. 150–178

The effect of heat, humidity and the body's thermoregulatory response on the respiratory system:

- Dehydration and drying of the airways in temperatures above 32°C makes breathing difficult, leading to:
  - increased mucus production
  - constriction of the airways
  - decreased volume of air for gaseous exchange.
- Increased breathing frequency to maintain oxygen consumption, leading to:
  - increased oxygen 'cost' of exercise.
- High levels of sunlight increase the effects of pollutants in the air, causing:
  - increased irritation of airways, leading to coughing, wheezing or asthma symptoms.

The overall effects of the thermal strain placed upon the cardiovascular and respiratory systems are increased oxygen 'cost' of activity and decreased aerobic energy production. This shifts more emphasis to anaerobic energy production, using carbohydrate (glycogen and glucose) stores more quickly. Exercise duration decreases as lactic acid accumulates readily, which results in early fatigue. Strength endurance and aerobic capacity are reduced, decreasing performance in mid- to long-distance events such as cycling, athletics and team games, such as football. Athletes with exercise-induced asthma must take precautions, using bronchodilators prior to dry heat exposure and staying adequately hydrated.

Effect on performance

When taking into account air temperature, solar radiation (from the sun), humidity and wind speed (wet-bulb globe temperature, WBGT), a precise picture of environmental conditions can be measured. Figure 1.2.11 shows the effects that increasingly hot environmental conditions have on marathon performance. For example, marathon runners finishing in 180 minutes (3 hours) may see a decrease in performance from 3 per cent at 10°C up to 12 per cent at 25°C. This would increase their finishing time to 185.4 minutes at 10°C and 201.6 minutes at 25°C. At higher temperatures, perceived exertion will feel harder for the athlete and performance times will be more severely affected.

Strength- and endurance-based physical activities and sports are affected differently in the heat and humidity due to the differing intensity, duration and opportunity for fluid intake. Interestingly, hyperthermia does not affect

Activity

Using Table 1.2.3, consider the metabolic heat produced by the trunk region compared with the muscle and skin both at rest and during strenuous exercise. Discuss the connection between your findings and the vascular shunt mechanism (redistribution of cardiac output). Extend your answer by considering how the increased blood flow to the skin for heat loss impairs the vascular shunt mechanism.

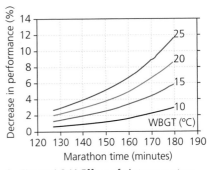

▲ Figure 1.2.11 Effect of air temperature, solar radiation, humidity and wind speed (WBGT) on marathon performance

maximal strength production, therefore many explosive and maximal events such as sprinting, throwing and jumping seem unaffected.

However, the longer the event, such as the marathon, the greater the effect on performance due to the gradual rise in heart and metabolic rate associated with increased core temperature. The more elite the long-distance runner, the lower the impact of heat and humidity due to physiological adaptations, precautions and heat acclimatisation. If an athlete or coach fails to understand the impact of heat and humidity on the body and performance, they may severely underestimate the effects and fatigue early in the race if the athlete's 'pace per mile' is not adjusted. Coaches of mid- to long-distance athletes competing in the heat and humidity can take steps to minimise the decrease in performance.

Pre competition:

- Acclimatise to increased temperatures. Seven to fourteen days of acclimatisation in the same conditions (naturally or within a thermal chamber) increases the body's tolerance to heat by:
  - increasing plasma volume, the onset and rate of sweating, and the efficiency of cardiac output distribution
  - decreasing the loss of electrolytes (salts and minerals that can conduct electrical impulses) within the sweat, which limits fatigue and cramping
  - decreasing heart rate at a given pace and temperature.
- Use cooling aids such as ice vests to reduce core temperature and delay the effect of high temperatures and dehydration.

During competition:

- Use pacing strategies to alter goals and reduce the feelings of exertion at low-exercise intensities.

▼ Table 1.2.4 An example of pacing strategies based on air temperature alone (runner at 8:00 min/mile pace)

Air temperature	Pace per mile	Impact
10°C	8:00 min/mile	None
16°C	8:12 min/mile	2–3% increase
21°C	8:31 min/mile	6–7% increase
27°C	9:06 min/mile	12–15% increase
29°C	9:31 min/mile	18–20% increase
Above 29°C	Listen to your body and use extreme caution.	

- Wear suitable clothing that maximises heat loss, removing sweat from the skin rapidly, such as lightweight compression wear.
- Rehydrate as often and as much as possible with a hypotonic or isotonic solution that replaces primarily lost fluids but also glucose and the electrolytes (salts) lost through the sweat.

Post competition:

- Cooling aids, such as cold towels and cold fans, aid the return of core body temperature gradually.
- Rehydrate using isotonic solutions that replace lost fluids, glucose and electrolytes.

According to experts, heatstroke is second only to head and spinal injuries as the number one cause of death in athletes. Common symptoms of heat stress in athletes include heat cramps, sharp pains in the muscles caused by a failure to replace the salts lost through the sweat. If untreated, heat exhaustion can follow. This is the significant loss of water and salt through excessive or prolonged sweating. Signs may include weakness, dizziness, visual disturbances, intense thirst, nausea, breathlessness, palpitations and numbness of the hands and feet. Recovery in a cool area with maximum rehydration supervised by a medical team is essential.

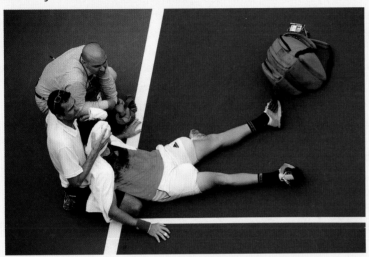

▲ Figure 1.2.12 Tennis player Jack Sock receives treatment for heat exhaustion in the 2015 US Open

Summary

- Understanding recovery is essential to plan training and competition correctly. Acclimatisation to the environmental conditions of an event is also essential to maintain peak performance. Recovery returns the body to a pre-exercise state using EPOC to continue aerobic energy production:
  - The fast component of recovery uses 1–4 litres of O_2 over three minutes to resaturate haemoglobin and myoglobin, repaying the oxygen deficit and generating energy to resynthesise ATP and PC stores.
  - The slow component of recovery uses 5–8 litres of O_2 over approximately 1–2 hours to generate energy to maintain ventilation, circulation and body temperature, remove carbon dioxide and lactic acid, and replenish glycogen stores.
- The implications of recovery on training are to include a warm up and active recovery, use cooling aids, use appropriate intensity and work:relief ratios and the correct nutrition.
- pO_2 in the atmospheric air decreases with increasing altitude, affecting the efficiency of the cardiovascular and respiratory systems. The diffusion gradient, rate of diffusion, O_2 saturation in the blood stream and delivery to the working muscles all decrease, limiting aerobic energy production. As a result, breathing frequency increases as blood and stroke volume decreases to reduce the intensity and duration of performance.
- Acclimatisation to altitude is the gradual adaptation to the lower pO_2 to reduce its negative effects. From 3–5 days up to 2 weeks' acclimatisation will increase erythropoietin and red blood cell production, stabilise breathing rate, reduce cardiac output and reduce the incidence of ill effects.
- Sustained sub-maximal exercise in hot and humid conditions causes the cardiovascular drift and potential dehydration:
  - Cardiovascular effects include increased blood flow to the skin and rate of sweating, decreased blood volume, venous return, stroke volume, cardiac output and blood pressure, reduced transport of O_2 and aerobic energy production.
  - Respiratory effects include drying, irritation and constriction of the airways, increased mucus production and breathing frequency, which increase the oxygen cost of activity.

1   Answer the following statements as true or false:
    a   EPOC is the volume of oxygen consumed post exercise to return the body to a pre-exercise state.
    b   Oxygen deficit is repayed during the slow lactacid stage of recovery.
    c   The fast alactacid stage of recovery uses 5–8 litres of O_2 and requires three minutes.
    d   Glyconeogenesis is the conversion of pyruvic acid into glycogen.
    e   Carbon dioxide can be removed in the plasma, as carbonic acid (H_2CO_3) and by combining with haemoglobin ($HbCO_2$).
    f   A work:relief ratio of 1:3 is best suited for lactate tolerance training.
    g   Coaches should use timeouts and substitutions to allow 30-second relief intervals for 50 per cent ATP and PC replenishment.
    h   An active recovery is essential for the removal of lactic acid from the muscles and blood stream.

2   Identify the key terms from the following statements:
    a   Height or elevation above sea level associated with a lower partial pressure of oxygen.
    b   A process undertaken to adapt to a change in environmental conditions.
    c   The bodily response to maintain internal core temperature.
    d   A loss of water in bodily tissues largely caused by sweating.
    e   An upward rise in heart rate during prolonged sub-maximal activity associated with an increase in body temperature.

Practice questions

1   Define the term 'excess post-exercise oxygen consumption' (EPOC) and explain the processes that occur during the slow, lactacid stage of recovery.   (6 marks)

2   Using a performer in a sport of your choice, describe the implications of recovery for a coach who is planning a training micro-cycle.   (8 marks)

3   Discuss the importance of acclimatisation and the timing of arrival for an aerobic event at an altitude over 2,400 m.   (6 marks)

4   Define the term 'cardiovascular drift' and explain the process of temperature regulation during exercise in the heat. Explain the effect of both the cardiovascular drift and temperature regulation on the efficiency of the cardiovascular system for an athlete performing a long-distance event in a hot and humid environment.   (20 marks)

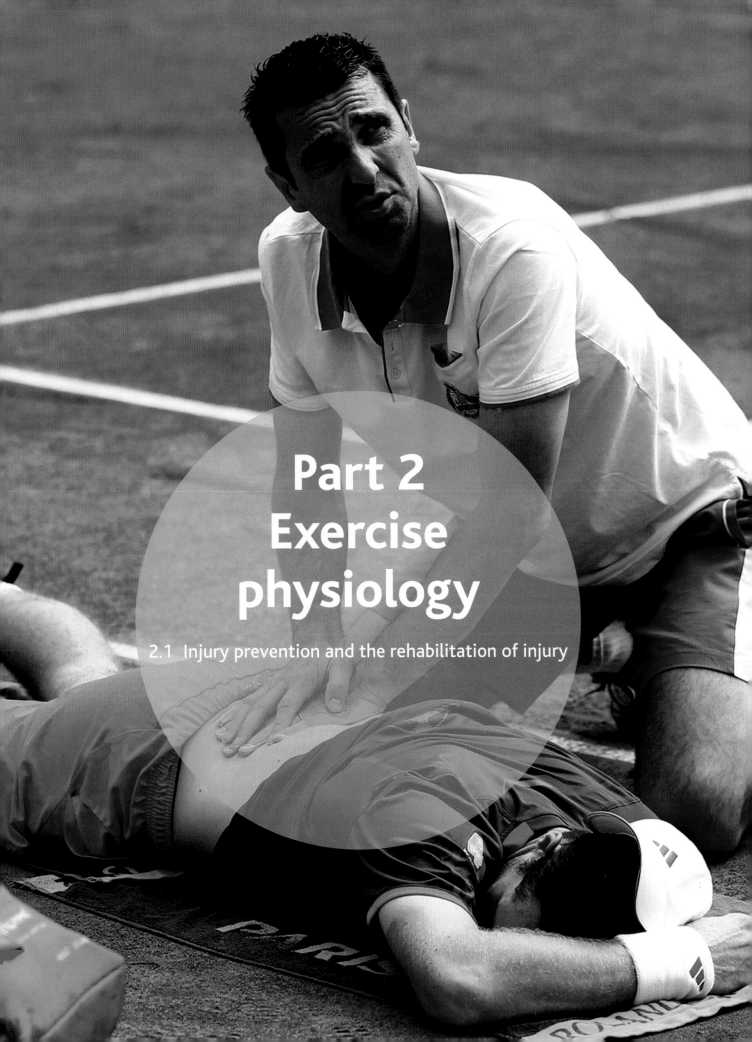

Part 2
Exercise
physiology

2.1 Injury prevention and the rehabilitation of injury

2.1 Injury prevention and the rehabilitation of injury

Understanding the specification

By the end of this chapter you should be able to demonstrate knowledge and understanding of acute and chronic injuries during physical activity and sport, injury prevention strategies, immediate response strategies and the rehabilitation of sports injuries.

Injuries:

- acute hard and soft tissue injuries
- concussion
- chronic hard and soft tissue injuries.

Injury prevention:

- intrinsic and extrinsic risk factors
- effectiveness of a warm up and a cool down.

Injury response:

- assessment using SALTAPS
- acute management using PRICE
- recognising concussion using the six Rs.

Injury rehabilitation:

- treatment methods: stretching, massage, heat, cold and contrast therapies, anti-inflammatory drugs, physiotherapy and surgery
- treatment of fractures, joint injuries and exercise-induced muscle damage.

Sports injuries account for many lost training hours and match performances per year and can cost an elite team tens of thousands of pounds if a player is ruled out for several months. Overtraining, lack of preparation, poor technique or impacts from a collision or fall can all cause injuries. Common sports injuries include strains and sprains in netball, fractures in football, dislocations in rugby, and tendinosis in tennis, golf and athletics.

Sports professionals play a significant part in injury prevention and rehabilitation, with roles such as strength and conditioning specialists, technical coaches, physiotherapists, sports massage therapists, orthopaedic surgeons and sports medicine specialists. There are many potential careers in this field working directly with elite athletes.

Acute and chronic injuries

There are two types of injury associated with physical activity and sport:

- **Acute injuries** occur at a specific moment in time, when there is a sudden injury associated with a traumatic event, such as a fracture of a bone in a boxer's jaw or a knee ligament tear after a bad tackle in football. Common causes of acute injuries are a collision between two players, a fall from a horse, or excessive impact from an object – for example, a football.

- **Chronic injuries** occur over a period of time. A chronic injury is a slowly developed injury associated with repeated or continuous stress or overuse, such as pain in a tennis player's elbow or a runner's heels. Common causes of chronic injuries are a sudden increase in the intensity, frequency or duration of activity, reduction in recovery, inadequate equipment or technique, poor range of motion, and an inadequate warm up and cool down.

Injuries are also classified as hard or soft, referring to the type of tissue damaged:

- **Hard tissue injuries** involve damage to the bone, joint or cartilage and include fractures and dislocations. Hard tissue injuries can result in internal bleeding, circulatory problems and joint instability and usually require hospital treatment.
- **Soft tissue injuries** are the most common in sport and include strains and sprains of the muscles, tendons or ligaments. Soft tissue injuries result in inflammation and bruising (internal bleeding) and require immediate attention to minimise recovery times.

Acute injuries

Acute injuries occur suddenly while participating in physical activity and can cause a lot of damage to bones, muscles, tendons and ligaments. Common examples are a football player fracturing a metatarsal when kicking a ball, a rugby player being tackled poorly and suffering anterior cruciate ligament (ACL) damage in the knee, and a netballer spraining her ankle in a bad landing. Signs and symptoms of an acute injury include sudden and severe pain, swelling, bruising, lack of movement or disfiguration.

Hard tissue injuries

Fractures

A **fracture** is a partial or complete break in a bone due to an excessive force that overcomes the bone's potential to flex. The fracture usually comes from a direct force (from a collision or object) or an indirect force (falling or poor technique). Common indications of a fracture are pain at the fracture site, inability to move or unnatural movement of the injured area, deformity, swelling and discoloration. All fractures are serious; however, the signs, symptoms, and length and type of treatment will depend on the type of fracture diagnosed:

- Compound (open) fractures: the fractured bones themselves break through the skin, creating an open wound with a high risk of infection.
- Simple (closed) fractures: the skin remains unbroken as the fracture causes little movement of the bone and therefore minimises the damage to the soft tissue surrounding it.

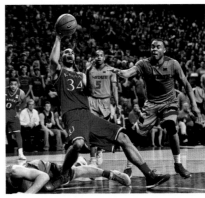

▲ Figure 2.1.1 Researchers have reported 20–40 per cent of acute ankle sprains lead to chronic problems

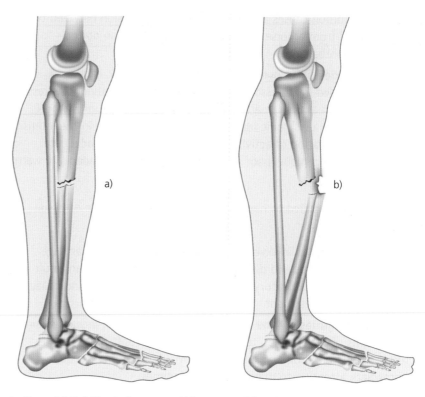

▲ Figure 2.1.2 a) Simple fracture and b) compound fracture

- Incomplete fracture: a partial crack in the bone that doesn't completely separate the bone.
- Complete fracture: a total break in the bone which separates the bone into one or more fragments.
- Greenstick fracture: a splitting partial break in the bone resulting from a bending action (just like a fresh twig).
- Transverse, oblique and spiral fractures: a crack perpendicular, diagonal or twisting diagonal respectively across the length of the bone.
- Comminuted fracture: a crack producing multiple fragments of bone and a long recovery process.
- Impacted fracture: a break caused by the ends of a bone being compressed together.
- Avulsion fracture: a bone fragment detached at the site of connective tissue attachment.

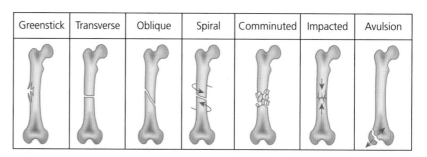

Greenstick	Transverse	Oblique	Spiral	Comminuted	Impacted	Avulsion

▲ Figure 2.1.3 Additional types of possible fracture

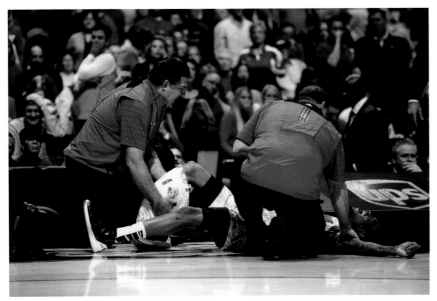

▲ Figure 2.1.4 Kevin Ware, a Georgia State University basketball player, suffered one of sport's most horrific open fractures on screen in 2013

Dislocation

A **dislocation** occurs when one bone is displaced from another, moving them out of their original position. A dislocation usually occurs from a direct force (from a collision or object) or an indirect force (a fall) pushing the joint past its extreme range of motion. Typical sites for dislocation are the shoulder, hip, knee, ankle, elbow, fingers and toes. Common indications of a dislocation are severe pain at the injury site, loss of movement, deformity, swelling, or a 'pop' feeling. All dislocations require treatment by a medical practitioner to ensure the bones are replaced in the correct alignment without causing further damage to the joint.

A **subluxation** (an incomplete or partial dislocation) often causes damage to the ligaments that connect bone to bone. When overstretched, ligaments can permanently lengthen, which decreases joint stability and increases the likelihood of recurrent dislocations. This may result in surgeries and compromise a long-term playing career.

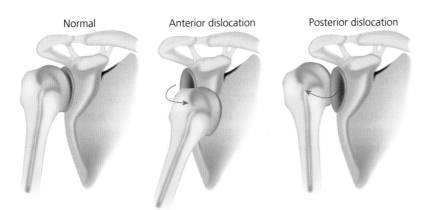

Normal   Anterior dislocation   Posterior dislocation

▲ Figure 2.1.5 Anterior and posterior dislocation of the humerus from the shoulder joint. The shoulder is vulnerable to dislocation due to the shallow socket and large range of motion

Key terms

Dislocation: the displacement of one bone from another out of their original position.
Subluxation: an incomplete or partial dislocation.

Activity

Research the injuries of the following footballers and consider whether the injuries affected their playing career:
- Petr Cech playing for Chelsea against Reading in 2006.
- Djibril Cisse playing for Liverpool against Blackburn Rovers in 2004 and then for France against China in 2006.
- Alan Smith playing for Manchester United against Liverpool in 2006.
- Kelly Smith captaining Arsenal Ladies against Sunderland in 2015.

Activity

Research the debate surrounding a call for tackling to be banned in school rugby. Focus on injuries, including fractures, dislocations and concussion.

Soft tissue injuries

Contusion and haematoma

A contusion, also known as a bruise, is an area of skin or tissue in which the blood vessels have **ruptured** (torn). Most contusions are minor and heal rapidly without a break in play or training. Severe contusions, however, can cause deep tissue damage, preventing participation in sport for months. Contusions are caused by a fall or direct impact from a player or object. They are second only to strains as an example of sports injury.

The damaged tissue leads to a **haematoma**: localised congealed bleeding from the ruptured blood vessels, which is relatively or totally confined to a tissue – for example, a muscle. Haematomas can range from superficial small bruises to deep bleeds that seep into surrounding tissues. Signs and symptoms include swelling and discoloration.

Key terms

Rupture: a complete tear of a muscle, tendon or ligament.
Haematoma: localised congealed bleeding from the ruptured blood vessels.

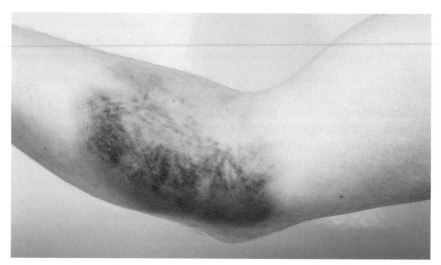

▲ Figure 2.1.6 A significant forearm haematoma

Sprain

Key term

Sprain: overstretch or a tear in the ligament that connects bone to bone.

A **sprain** is damage (overstretch or tear) to the ligaments which connect bone to bone and support a joint. It is usually caused by a sudden twist, impact or fall that forces the joint beyond its extreme range of motion. Sprains most commonly occur to the ankle of games players and athletes, but also to the knees of footballers and skiers and the thumbs and wrist of an athlete bracing a fall.

Signs and symptoms of a sprain include pain, swelling, bruising, inability to bear weight and possible dislocation. The severity of a sprain ranges from overstretch of a few ligament fibres (first-degree sprain) to a partial tear (second-degree sprain), a total rupture (tear) or detachment of a ligament from the bone (third-degree sprain).

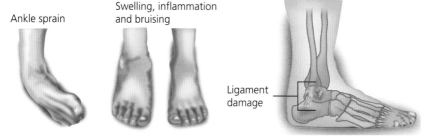

Ankle sprain

Swelling, inflammation and bruising

Ligament damage

▲ Figure 2.1.7 Signs and symptoms of an ankle sprain

Strain

A **strain** is damage (overstretch or tear) to the muscle fibres or tendon connecting muscle to bone. It is usually caused by overstretching a particular area or contracting muscle fibres too quickly, resulting in overstretch, and partial or complete rupture of the muscle fibres or tendon. Strains most commonly occur in sports that involve dynamic lunging and explosive movements, such as lunging to return a drop shot in badminton and sprinting out of the blocks in the 100 m, and contact activities such as tackling in football.

Signs and symptoms of a strain include pain on movement, swelling and discoloration or bruising. The severity of a strain ranges from minor damage to the fibres (grade 1), to more extensive damage but not completely ruptured (grade 2), to a complete rupture (grade 3), which will require surgery and significant rehabilitation.

Abrasion

An **abrasion** is superficial damage to the skin caused by a scraping action against a playing surface, such as falling or slipping on an athletics track, netball court or artificial surface, or clothing rubbing on the body, such as chafing during a marathon. If the abrasion causes an open wound, it may contain dirt or gravel and require cleaning. If a laceration (cut) is caused, medical attention may be required for suturing (stitching).

Most sports now have blood rules requiring the player to leave the game until the bleeding stops, irrespective of the size of the injury. For example, in netball the presence of blood requires an official to stop the game and allow two minutes to stem the flow and decide whether the player is fit to continue.

Blisters

Blisters are the separation of layers of skin where a pocket of fluid forms due to friction. Although painful, they may not stop participation with treatment and they are preventable with the correct equipment, footwear and training load.

Key terms

Strain: overstretch or tear in the muscle or tendon that connects muscle to bone.
Abrasion: superficial damage to the skin caused by a scraping action against a surface.
Blister: friction forming separation of layers of skin where a pocket of fluid forms.

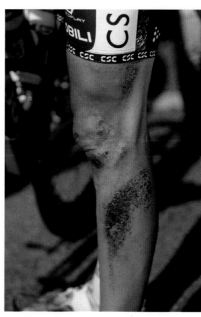

▲ Figure 2.1.8 Old and new abrasions on a cyclist's leg

Activity

Fill in the blanks in the following paragraph:
A _____ is damage to the ligaments whereas a _____ is damage to the muscle or tendons. A _____ is associated with overstretching an area or contracting muscle fibres too rapidly whereas a _____ is associated with a twist, impact or fall. A _____ is common in games players such as in netball and rugby whereas a _____ is common in explosive athletes such as sprinting and badminton players.

Concussion

Key term

Concussion: a traumatic brain injury resulting in a disturbance of brain function.

Concussion is a traumatic brain injury resulting in a disturbance of brain function, such as headaches, dizziness, balance problems, nausea, and in around 10 per cent of cases a loss of consciousness. Concussion can be caused by a direct blow to the head or blows to other parts of the body, which cause rapid movement of the head and therefore can be common in sports such as boxing, rugby, football and horse racing.

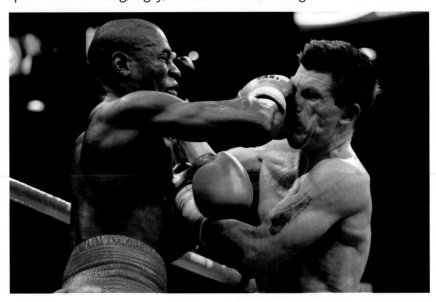

▲ Figure 2.1.9 Concussion is a regular occurrence in boxing and stars can suffer the effects years later

Activity

Research the 'George North incident' when, during a Wales vs England Six Nations (2015) match, player George North received two significant blows to the head but remained on the pitch. After researching the evidence, do you agree with the decisions made?

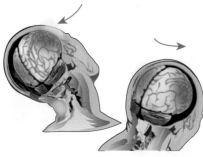

▲ Figure 2.1.10 The force from a blow to the head causes the brain to hit the inner surface of the skull and rebound against the other side

The jelly-like brain floats in cerebrospinal fluid within the skull. On impact the blow to the head accelerates the brain against the rough inner wall of the skull and then rebounds back against the other side. This can cause swelling and a disruption in the biochemistry and electrical processes between the neurons in the brain, which leads to the confusion-like symptoms of a mild brain injury. If a concussion or suspected concussion has occurred, it is essential that the player is removed from play and seen by a healthcare professional. If in doubt, sit it out!

Activity

Research the issue of concussion in American football. How does the high-impact nature of the game influence the rules, regulation and incidence of concussion?

IN THE NEWS

Concussion is a serious issue on the rugby pitch and in 2013–14 it was the most common injury for the third consecutive season, with 86 match concussions accounting for 12.4 per cent of all match injuries. On average there are 10.5 concussions per 1,000 playing hours compared with 17 in boxing and 25 in jump horse racing. The Rugby Football Union (RFU), in partnership with Oxford University, is aiming to recruit 40 per cent of the England Retired Internationals Club (ERIC) to launch a study into how rugby has affected their cognitive function and musculoskeletal system to gain an understanding of the long-term consequences of an international rugby career.

▼ Table 2.1.1 Symptoms of concussion in sport

Symptoms clearly indicate concussion	Symptoms may indicate concussion
Post-traumatic seizure Loss of consciousness Balance problems Disorientation and confusion Dazed or blank expression	Lying motionless Slow to get up Grabbing or clutching head Headache Dizziness Visual problems Nausea or vomiting Fatigue Light sensitivity

RESEARCH IN FOCUS

Archbold *et al.* conducted rugby injury surveillance in Ulster schools and published findings in the *British Journal of Sports Medicine* in 2015. Looking at 825 players over one playing season, they found 426 injuries, with more than 50 per cent occurring in a tackle or collision situation. 36.8 per cent of players suffered at least one injury, with 49 per cent resulting in absence for more than 28 days. Concussion accounted for the most significant time out of play (15.9 per cent), followed by shoulder dislocation (10.6 per cent), knee sprain (9.1 per cent), ankle sprain (6.7 per cent) and hand injury (5.3 per cent). The researchers concluded there was a higher risk of injury with greater age, weight and playing standard.

Chronic injuries resulting from continuous stress to the body

Chronic injuries occur over a period of time while participating in physical activity and are often referred to as overuse injuries due to the repeated or continuous stress placed on a specific part of the body. Common examples are stress fractures along the tibia of basketball players, **osteoarthritis** in the knees of skiers, Achilles tendinopathy in runners' heels, and tennis elbow after repetitive motion. Signs and symptoms of a chronic injury include pain when participating, swelling after each activity, and small, nagging aches in a specific area when at rest. Although the symptoms are milder than acute injuries, if left untreated they can grow into a debilitating injury that impacts on daily life.

Hard tissue injuries

Stress fracture

A **stress fracture** is a tiny crack in the surface of a bone, usually caused by fatigued muscles transferring their stress overload to the bone tissue. It is an overuse injury that is sometimes referred to as a fatigue or insufficiency fracture. Specific spots of pain during physical activity may indicate a stress fracture; however, the pain subsides with rest, and using a typical X-ray, stress fractures are hard to spot.

Stress fractures are common in distance running, tennis, gymnastics and basketball players, where the repetitive stress of the foot on the ground without sufficient rest periods can cause trauma. Most stress fractures occur in the lower body and fractures of the tibia are most common. Overtraining, intensity overload, unfamiliar surfaces and inappropriate equipment all contribute to stress fractures.

> **Key term**
>
> **Osteoarthritis:** degeneration of articular cartilage from the bone surfaces within a joint, causing pain and restricted movement.

> **Key term**
>
> **Stress fracture:** a tiny crack in the surface of a bone caused by overuse.

41

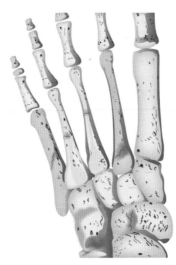

▲ Figure 2.1.11 Metatarsal stress fractures

Key term

Bone spurs: outgrowths of bone into a joint, causing pain and restricted movement.

Activity

Osteoarthritis is the most common form of joint disease, caused by the breakdown and loss of articular cartilage from the bone surfaces within a joint. Joints swell and underlying bone thickens and forms rough spurs (**bone spurs**), making movement painful and severely restricted. Research the causes of osteoarthritis and discuss whether it could be classed as a chronic hard tissue 'injury'. Extend your research to consider former Arsenal goalkeeping legend Bob Wilson linking osteoarthritis to previous acute injuries.

Soft tissue injuries

Shin splints

'**Shin splints**' is a term used to describe chronic shin pain. As a result of repeated overuse the tibialis anterior (anterior shin splints) and tibialis posterior (posterior shin splints) can become injured through excessive loading stress, resulting in tenderness and inflammation, especially in the morning as muscles stiffen overnight. The tendons connecting muscle to the shin bone attach on the outer casing of the bone known as the periosteum. In almost all cases of shin splints the connection between the tendon and periosteum becomes inflamed, leading to pain in specific areas of the shin bone. There are several closely related conditions affecting the muscles, tendons and bone surfaces; however, the most common form of shin splints is also known as **medial tibial stress syndrome (MTSS)**.

MTSS has been frequently reported by distance runners, dancers, football players, gymnasts and army recruits and is largely caused by overuse and overtraining on hard or uneven surfaces. Runners often suffer shin splints at the beginning of training by doing 'too much, too soon' or abruptly changing training routines. Being overweight, wearing inadequate footwear and poor leg biomechanics can also lead to shin splints.

Tendinosis

A tendon is a tough band of fibrous (around 86 per cent collagen) connective tissue that connects muscle to bone. It is designed to transmit forces and withstand stress during muscular contraction. **Tendinosis** is the deterioration of a tendon's collagen in response to chronic overuse.

Key terms

Shin splints/medial tibial stress syndrome (MTSS): chronic shin pain due to the inflammation of muscles and stress on the tendon attachments to the surface of the tibia.

Tendinosis: the deterioration of a tendon in response to chronic overuse and repetitive strain.

Repetitive strain causes small-scale injuries that are not given the time to heal and so accumulate, resulting in a chronic injury. Signs and symptoms of tendinosis are burning, stinging, aching, tenderness and stiffness, common in the wrist, forearm, elbow, shoulder, knee or heel.

Athletes performing repetitive movements without the appropriate rest periods between training may develop tendinosis, such as:

- **Achilles tendinosis**: pain, tightness and deterioration in the tendon behind the ankle common in distance runners; a slow progression of pain which will lead to difficulty climbing stairs or running

- **tennis elbow** (lateral epicondylitis): strenuous overuse of the tendons in the forearm during repeated twisting actions can lead to microscopic tears, pain and tightness that limit movement; common in athletes who overtrain in racket sports or throwing activities.

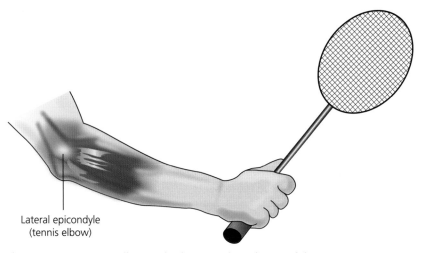

Lateral epicondyle (tennis elbow)

▲ Figure 2.1.12 Tennis elbow is also known as lateral epicondylitis

Extend your knowledge

Another overuse injury is bursitis, a painful condition that affects small, fluid-filled sacs that cushion bones, tendons and muscles near your joints. As with all chronic overuse injuries, bursitis occurs in joints performing repetitive motions and is relieved only by proper rest and recuperation.

Activity

Among your class, friends or family, discuss previous sporting injuries. Classify the type of injury: whether acute or chronic, hard tissue or soft.

Activity

Categorise the following injuries as either acute or chronic and hard or soft tissue:

	Acute injury	Chronic injury	Hard tissue	Soft tissue
Concussion				
Complete fracture				
Tennis elbow				
Sprain				
Stress fracture				
Tendinosis				
Strain				
Shin splints				

Below is a table of sports and their typical injury profile.

Sport	Common injuries
Athletics	Muscle strain to the legs and lower back due to explosive movements Ankle sprain and strain due to dynamic and repetitive movements Achilles tendinosis due to repeated movements Stress fractures in repetitive jump athletes
Cricket	Head fractures and concussion due to fast bowling Strains in a bowler's back due to awkward repetitive movement pattern Knee sprain and strain due to dynamic movement and repetitive twisting
Football	Metatarsal fractures due to high-impact kicking Abrasions and boot-stud injuries in tackling Knee and ankle sprain and strain due to dynamic movement and repetitive twisting
Racket sports	Tennis elbow due to repetitive movements Fractures due to falling on hard surfaces Muscle strain injury through repetitive movement Tendonitis or tendon inflammation in the shoulder due to repeated overhead movements

Injury prevention

Sporting injuries constitute a threat to athletes' health and in some cases can lead to permanent disability. Studies have found up to 19 per cent of all acute injuries seen in accident and emergency departments are linked to sports participation, with 15–25 year olds and females at most risk. Athletes performing dynamic high-impact, contact and repetitive action sports such as basketball, football, rugby and athletics seem highly at risk.

The risk factors must be identified and minimised in a bid to prevent injuries. This will maximise training and performance quality and prevent lengthy breaks in training or competition for injury rehabilitation. Risk factors have two classifications:

- **Intrinsic risk factors** are risks or forces from within the body:
  - aspects of an athlete's physical make-up or individual variables, such as poor posture and alignment, previous injury and insufficient nutrition
  - training effects, such as inappropriate flexibility, strength imbalance and poor preparation for training.
- **Extrinsic risk factors** are risks or forces from outside the body:
  - poor biomechanical training and performance techniques
  - incorrect equipment and clothing
  - inappropriate overload without progression and lack of variance in training.

Key terms

Intrinsic injury risk factor: an injury risk or force from inside the body.
Extrinsic injury risk factor: an injury risk or force from outside the body.

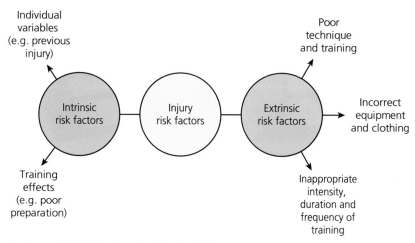

▲ Figure 2.1.13 Intrinsic and extrinsic risk factors

Intrinsic risk factors

Individual variables

There are many factors that contribute to injury risk within an athlete's make-up which need to be taken into account when training and performing:

● Previous injury is the biggest risk factor for soft tissue injury and an athlete should never return to training after an injury until declared fit to do so. Injuries can cause a loss in connective tissue strength, imbalance between muscle groups, decreased joint stability, altered biomechanics, a deficit in neuromuscular function and proprioception.

● Posture and alignment issues, such as different leg lengths, scoliosis (lateral curvature of the spine) or lordosis (inward curvature of the spine), cause biomechanical changes requiring connective tissues to handle forces in unnatural ways. This increases the risk of injury. For example, the International Olympic Congress on Sports and Dance stated the most common cause of dance injury to lower legs, ankles and feet was dancers' failure to keep their feet and legs aligned naturally. A small misalignment causes joints to weaken and leads to a muscular imbalance in the lower leg and foot.

● Age increases injury risk as bone tissue loses strength and as connective tissues suffer overuse, wear and tear they become more prone to injury.

● Nutrition is important for injury prevention and also for recovery: protein for growth and repair of cells and tissues and collagen formation, carbohydrates for energy production to reduce the onset of fatigue, fats for protection and cushioning, and vitamins and minerals, such as vitamin D and calcium, for bone growth and repair.

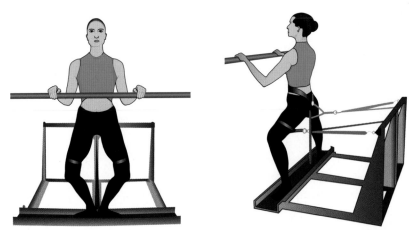

▲ Figure 2.1.14 Specially designed equipment to maintain the correct posture and alignment for dancers at the barre

RESEARCH IN FOCUS

Fulton *et al.* published a review of injury risk research in the *International Journal for Sports Physical Therapy* in 2014 (9(5): 583–595) and concluded:

- hamstring strain was 4.3–11.6 times more likely in those with a previous hamstring strain than those without

- anterior cruciate ligament (ACL) injury occurred on the same leg as previous ACL in up to 70 per cent of cases in elite footballers

- ankle sprain was 21–50 per cent higher in those with a previous ankle sprain.

View this open access paper titled 'Injury risk is altered by previous injury: a systematic review of the literature and presentation of causative neuromuscular factors' and discuss the range of studies, study populations and risk factors. (Go to the PubMed website: www.ncbi. nlm.nih.gov/pubmed and using the search feature enter the title of the research paper above.)

Training effects

There are many factors over which an athlete can have a level of control to prepare appropriately for training and performance:

- Poor preparation will increase the risk of injury. Running a marathon without the appropriate training will result in potentially catastrophic injury. The correct warm up, nutrition, hydration, sleep, training and fitness level are essential for the intensity, duration and frequency of activity undertaken.

- Inadequate fitness levels can lead to injury if the intensity, duration or frequency of training or ability of opponents are too high. Early fatigue can lead to poor technique, wrong decisions and a drop in performance, which increase the risk of injury.

- Inappropriate flexibility level can lead to poor joint stability. A lack of flexibility in the connective tissues can limit range of motion and lead to acute sprain and strain injuries. An appropriate warm up with sport-specific mobility exercises may increase performance while limiting injury risk. Too much flexibility can also lead to poor joint stability and collision injuries may lead to dislocations.

Extrinsic risk factors

Poor technique and training

Overuse injuries are largely caused by performing repetitive actions with poor biomechanical technique. Excessive stress will be placed on muscles, tendons and ligaments, which over time can deteriorate; for example, tennis elbow is often associated with poor backhand technique. Poor technique can also cause acute injuries. Poor technique when lifting and handling equipment such as exercise machines can lead to muscle strains, while poor tackling technique in rugby can lead to a potential concussion. Poor technique will also limit strength, power and speed when performing specific movements.

Coaches play a critical role in injury prevention by teaching the correct technique, warm up routines and practices appropriate for the age and ability of their players. A coach should be qualified and responsible for keeping up to date with new training guidelines and match rules to enhance the safety of the players. For example:

- Rugby has seen many rule changes and adaptations to reduce the potential for injury, such as the 'scrum engagement sequence' to reduce the inconsistency when waiting to engage. A rugby coach must communicate new rules and the modified rules for touch and sevens age groups to lower the risk of injury.

- An aerobics coach taking a step class must make sure participants use the correct height step and wear the proper footwear, use the appropriate speed of music and choreograph routines appropriate for the ability of participants.

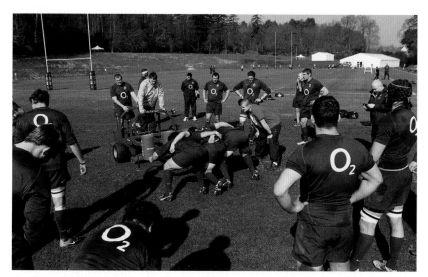

▲ Figure 2.1.15 England Rugby Union training session with expert coaching

Incorrect equipment and clothing

Equipment used in sport should be age, stature and ability related. Incorrect equipment could lead to or accelerate the onset of injury. For example, a child starting tennis should not use a full-size racket as the forces placed upon the connective tissues and joints will be excessive and unmanageable:

- Mini tennis, an adaptation by the Lawn Tennis Association, uses a smaller court, racket, net and a lower-bouncing ball to help to reduce the risk of acute and chronic injuries on the growing skeleton.

- Rugby Union regulations stipulate that equipment manufacturers must be approved by World Rugby and equipment must be fit for purpose. Training equipment includes senior and junior tackle bags, tackle shields, full body armour, contact tops and body wedges, all used to perfect technique while reducing the risk of injury.

Athletes can wear protective equipment to minimise the risk of injury to vulnerable parts of the body. This equipment should be age and size appropriate, follow sporting regulations and be checked for damage frequently. For example:

- tennis players opt for shoulder straps and netballers and basketballers wear ankle braces to add stability to a joint and minimise the risk of strain and sprains
- cricket batsmen wear knee guards to protect the patella (kneecap) and cartilage from acute injuries and helmets to minimise the risk of concussion
- boxers wear gum shields, gloves and sometimes head guards to minimise the risk of fracture or concussion
- winter sports athletes wear helmets, wrist guards, shin guards and sometimes braced clothing to minimise the risk of acute injuries such as fracture when hitting slalom poles or falling on the snow or ice.

Athletes must wear sport-specific clothing to maximise performance while reducing the risk of injury. Technological fabrics can:

- be a second skin – flexible for gymnasts and dancers to maximise range of motion and smooth to minimise air resistance for cyclists and skiers, thus limiting fatigue
- wick away moisture – aiding thermoregulation and preventing heat exhaustion in long-distance events
- be lightweight – layers to wick moisture, insulate and smooth can maintain the range of motion about a joint while preventing hypothermia (low core body temperature) in winter and mountain sports
- contain padding – reducing the impact of external forces in contact sports such as American football to protect the shoulder girdle from fractures and dislocations.

Footwear is designed for the demands of the sport, the specific athlete and the playing surface; for example, distance running shoes require cushioning for shock absorption, basketball shoes require lateral ankle support, fell running shoes require deep grips and little cushioning whereas indoor squash shoes have a shallow grip for maximum court contact. Generic trainers will lack the support necessary to balance body weight and cater for the explosive, dynamic or endurance nature of most sports, increasing the risk of injury, specifically acute ankle strain and sprains.

Inappropriate intensity, duration or frequency of activity

The principles of training must be followed when designing a training programme to ensure the risk of injury is minimised. Progressive overload ensures the athlete is pushed beyond their comfort zone to force an adaptation; however, the stress placed upon the body must be appropriate

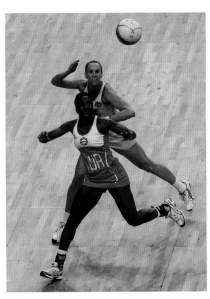

▲ Figure 2.1.16 An England netballer wears protective ankle braces to minimise the risk of injury

for the individual's age, ability, stature and injury status. This stress must be gradually increased to push adaptation and improvement but not compromise health and well-being:

- If the intensity of training is too great, acute injuries may occur as the forces placed upon the connective tissues and joints may be excessive.
- If the frequency or duration of training is too great, acute inflammatory injuries may occur, such as tendonitis, or chronic overuse injuries, such as stress fractures or tendinosis, may develop.
- If training methods used do not include a variety of activities and rest intervals, repetitive strain and overuse injuries may develop.

Activity

Classify the following football injuries by intrinsic or extrinsic risk factor:

1 Steven Gerrard in the 2011–12 season: hamstring and groin strain after an early return from previous injury.
2 Wayne Rooney: fifth metatarsal fracture after a bad tackle by Paulo Ferreira in 2006.
3 Nemanja Vidic: ACL sprain after using the improper tackling technique, falling and twisting his knee in 2011.
4 Fernando Torres: arguable overtraining and hamstring injuries in the 2008–09 season.
5 Eduardo da Silva: fibula fracture and ankle dislocation after his planted foot was caught by defender Martin Taylor in 2008.
6 Kelly Smith: worsening a stress fracture in 2012 on a video shoot while not wearing protective football boots.

Warm up and cool down effectiveness

A warm up and cool down are an essential part of every training session to minimise the risk of injury during the activity and maximise recovery after the activity. Although their usefulness is rarely challenged, the most effective form of warm up and cool down has been debated and will depend on the activity being performed.

Warm up

A warm up is performed to raise body temperature and prepare an athlete physiologically and psychologically for an activity to minimise the risk of injury and maximise performance. Research suggests an ideal warm up:

- lasts 20–45 minutes
- gradually increases in intensity
- has three distinct stages:
  - HR-raising activity to increase temperature, blood flow, HR, breathing frequency and O_2 delivery to the muscles
  - stretching and mobility exercises to lubricate and mobilise joints and increase the elasticity in connective tissues
  - sport-specific drills to activate neural pathways and rehearse movement patterns.

A rise in temperature of around 2–3° increases enzyme activity, diffusion gradients and metabolic activity, which improves the efficiency of muscular contraction. The elasticity of muscles, tendons and ligaments increases while antagonistic co-ordination improves, decreasing the risk of injury, such as sprain and strain.

Historically, static stretches have been a large part of warm up routines; for example, holding a biceps brachii stretch for 10 s in a bid to relax and lengthen connective tissues before performance. However, research suggests static stretching:

- has no effect on injury prevention
- may reduce the peak force produced in the Achilles tendon by 8 per cent
- deteriorates antagonistic co-ordination, hampering explosive movements
- reduces eccentric strength by 9 per cent, decreasing the ability to change direction at speed
- reduces a muscle's ability to consume O_2 by up to 50 per cent.

As a result, static stretching should be avoided in a warm up routine unless expressly advised by a physiotherapist, perhaps due to previous injury or scar tissue accumulation.

Injury prevention researchers believe the most effective connective tissue is warm, can cope with elastic or explosive strength, and is prepared for sudden dynamic loads. This requires dynamic flexibility stretches in sport-specific patterns – for example, squats, walking lunges and high knee skips – gradually increasing the reach, complexity and speed of the stretch. These exercises will include acceleration, deceleration, changes of direction, side-to-side (lateral) movement, balance and co-ordination exercises.

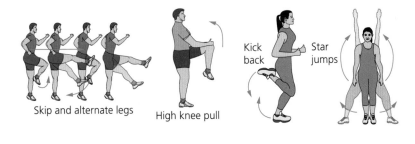

Skip and alternate legs

High knee pull

Kick back

Star jumps

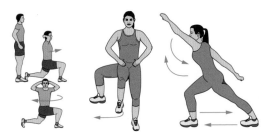

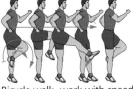

Bicycle walk, work with speed
Feet should pass over knees
Alternate legs

▲ Figure 2.1.17 Dynamic stretching exercises

Sports scientists in conjunction with physiotherapists and physicians have created specialist warm up programmes to reduce injury risk in athletes. FIFA's 11+ programme, ACTIVATE GAA and Prevent Injury and Enhance Performance (PEP) warm up programmes have been specially designed with:
- running, cutting and landing mechanics drills
- strength, plyometrics and balance work
- agility and power drills.

Using a specialised warm up programme during training and before a match for approximately three months significantly reduces acute and chronic lower leg and knee injury risk in games players.

Activity

Research the Sports Institute for Northern Ireland's ACTIVATE GAA programme. Set up this specialised warm up routine and discuss any differences to your normal warm up as part of a practical lesson or coaching session.

Cool down

A cool down (also termed active recovery) is performed to maintain heart rate, blood flow and metabolic activity to flush the muscle tissue with oxygenated blood, thus removing waste products and starting the healing process. An active cool down typically:

- lasts 20–30 minutes
- gradually decreases in intensity
- has several distinct stages:
  - moderate-intensity activity around 45–55 per cent of VO_2max to maintain HR, venous return mechanisms and blow flow to remove waste products from the muscle tissue
  - stretching exercises to reduce muscle tension, increase muscle relaxation and gradually lower the muscle temperature.

A cool down is just as important as a warm up to exercise recovery and injury prevention. Without a cool down, toxins and lactic acid build up, blood pools and levels of circulating adrenaline and endorphins cause restlessness and poor sleep. During high-intensity events with multiple heats or matches on the same day – for example, a one-day netball tournament with seven-minute matches – an active cool down has been proven far more beneficial than a passive (resting) recovery. The speed of lactic acid removal is increased and aerobic energy production is activated earlier, enhancing future performances, delaying fatigue and preventing fatigue-related injuries.

Historically, an active cool down has been thought beneficial for all sports; however, during low-intensity aerobic activity, such as jogging for an aerobically fit athlete, a passive recovery period (for example, sitting on a bench) has been shown to be beneficial, returning temperature and metabolic activity more quickly. Equally, there is little evidence to suggest an active cool down can prevent or limit **delayed onset muscle soreness (DOMS)**. DOMS is caused by micro-injury to the muscle fibres and requires time to heal, symptoms to subside and muscle fibres to adapt to the new stresses placed upon them. Soreness will peak 24–72 hours post heavy and eccentric exercise, such as plyometrics, and new training programmes or dramatic increases in intensity should be avoided.

Key term

Delayed onset muscle soreness (DOMS): pain and stiffness felt in the muscle, which peaks 24–72 hours after exercise, associated with eccentric muscle contractions.

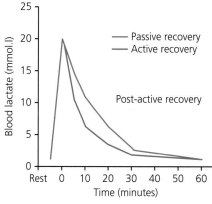

▲ Figure 2.1.18 Blood lactate removal rates during an active and a passive recovery period

Ankle injuries account for around 80 per cent of all injuries in netball and ankle sprains are the most common lower limb injury at 42 per cent. With most ankle sprains occurring on landing, fatigue can be a big risk factor. With fatigue, neuromuscular control may decrease, causing a lack of preparation for ankle stability. Injury prevention in netball should include:

- assessment of stability, balance and co-ordination
- regular training and match play
- netball-specific warm up drills that include jumping, landing and rapid change of direction
- ankle guards and supports for repetitive ankle sprains
- advice and support from a physiotherapist and strength and conditioning coach.

Responding to injuries and medical conditions in sport

Assessment using 'SALTAPS'

In a sporting event it is likely you may have seen an accident take place or have a particular understanding of the specific body part that has been injured. To consider whether a player should continue in the game or training, a close inspection using a sports-specific assessment such as **SALTAPS** will be useful:

- **S**top
  - Stop the game if a player is injured and observe the injury.
- **A**sk
  - Ask questions about the injury, such as where does it hurt, what type of pain is it, which way did you fall?
- **L**ook
  - Search for specific signs such as bruising, swelling, broken skin, bleeding or foreign objects.
- **T**ouch
  - Gently palpate the injured area to identify painful regions and inflammation.
- **A**ctive movement
  - Ask the player whether they can move the injured area without your assistance.
- **P**assive movement
  - If there is active movement, gently move the injured area through its full range of motion.
- **S**trength testing
  - Ask the player to stand, lift or put pressure on the injured area if they can. Ask them whether they feel able to continue playing and, if so, observe their movement and behaviour closely.

With the increasing intensity and risk associated with modern sports it is important to use this method with caution and stop at the appropriate stage for the injury.

Key term

SALTAPS: protocol for the assessment of a sporting injury: stop, ask, look, touch, active movement, passive movement and strength testing.

- If at the 'Look' stage there are obvious signs of injury, the player should be removed from the game or stop training to receive treatment. Equally, if the player is unconscious or there is a suspected neck or spinal injury, there should be no attempt to move the player.
- For the 'Touch, Active and Passive movement' stages it is important that the most qualified and experienced individual makes the assessment for an accurate account of the location, severity and type of injury.

Acute management using PRICE

Acute soft tissue injuries trigger inflammation, bruising and pain and can cause further damage if not treated quickly. The **PRICE** protocol has five simple steps that aim to minimise muscle or joint injury. When used immediately after an injury has occurred, swelling is reduced, pain is eased and further damage is prevented:

- **P**rotection
  - Protect the injury and the person from any further damage. Stop playing and use padding, splints or crutches to get off the field of play.
- **R**est
  - Allow the injury time to heal and prevent further damage – playing on can complicate injuries and increase recovery time.
- **I**ce
  - Apply ice indirectly to the skin to reduce inflammation and pain. General guidelines recommend 10 minutes of ice application which can be repeated after a 60-minute break.
- **C**ompression
  - Compressing the injury with tear tape, crepe or a stretch bandage will help to reduce swelling. Monitor the tightness of the compression as continued swelling can occur.
- **E**levation
  - Raise the injury above heart level to reduce blood flow to the area, thus decreasing swelling.

Most minor soft tissue injuries can be managed at home. For the first two to three days after your injury, you should follow the **PRICE** procedure.

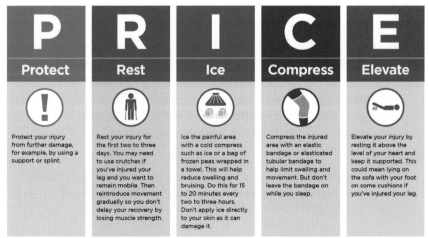

▲ Figure 2.1.19 Bupa's guide to PRICE

Activity

With a partner, imagine a scenario in your chosen sport where a player suddenly drops to the ground, clutches their lower leg and shouts in pain. Using the SALTAPS protocol, consider the type, severity and location (knee, shin, ankle or toes) of any potential injuries. Also consider with each injury the point at which you would stop the SALTAPS protocol.

Key term

PRICE: protocol for the treatment of acute injuries: protection, rest, ice, compression and elevation.

The PRICE protocol is the preferred method for immediate treatment of acute muscle strain injuries; however, its use is debated for acute ligament sprain injuries. The PRICE protocol decreases blood flow and immune response to the injured area, actually delaying collagen formation, range of motion and speed of recovery. Unlike muscles, ligaments have very few blood vessels, which reduces blood and nutrient supply and therefore delays healing. Alternative protocols that encourage movement and exercise with a course of pain relievers and physiotherapy may be the more preferred route.

Key term

Concussion six Rs: protocol for recognition of concussion: recognise, remove, refer, rest, recover and return.

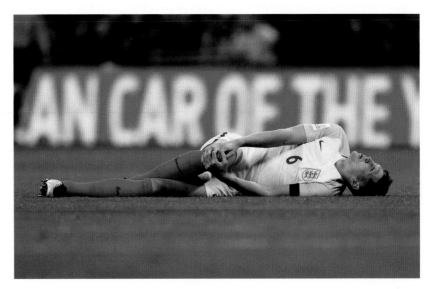

▲ Figure 2.1.20 FIFA states the PRICE regime can minimise the effects of muscle or joint injury

Recognising concussion using the 'six Rs'

Concussion is a brain injury and very serious. Concussion can be fatal and World Rugby (formerly the IRB) has launched a 'recognise and remove' campaign which involves **six Rs** to make sure most players can recover with just physical and mental rest:

- **R**ecognise
  - Parents, players, coaches and officials should all be aware of the signs and symptoms of concussion.
- **R**emove
  - If a player has a concussion or suspected concussion, they must be removed from the field of play immediately.
- **R**efer
  - If removed from the field the player should be referred immediately to a qualified healthcare professional who is trained in evaluating and treating concussion.
- **R**est
  - Players must rest from exercise until symptom free and not be left alone for the first 24 hours.
- **R**ecover
  - Players must fully recover and be symptom free before considering a return to play. Adults must take a minimum of one week and under-18s two weeks before seeking an authorised return from a healthcare professional. Rest and specific treatment through recovery are essential for the health of the injured participant.
- **R**eturn
  - To complete a safe return to the field the player must be symptom free, have written authorisation and complete the 'graduated return to play' protocol.

World Rugby's graduated return to play (GRTP) programme incorporates a progressive exercise protocol that introduces a player back to sport in a graded fashion:

1 Minimum rest period with complete body and brain rest without symptoms.
2 Light aerobic exercise to increase heart rate.
3 Sport-specific exercise incorporating running drills without any head impact.
4 Non-contact training drills with growing complexity to increase the cognitive load.
5 Full-contact practice with normal training activities to assess functional skills.
6 Return to play.

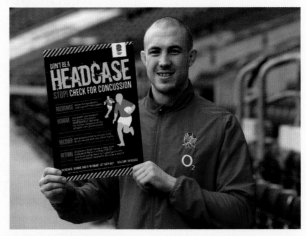

Figure 2.1.21 World Rugby #RecogniseAndRemove campaign for concussion awareness

Activity

Research the most common injuries in your chosen sport. Using your knowledge, understanding and research, create a poster summarising injury statistics, classification of injuries, potential causes and preventative methods that can be taken.

Rehabilitation of injury

Rehabilitation is the process undertaken to regain full function after an injury has occurred. A rehabilitation and strengthening programme is essential for full recovery and to prevent further injuries. It involves restoring strength, flexibility, endurance and speed in the connective tissues in a bid for an athlete to return to training and perform as quickly as possible. If an injured performer returns to training or competition too early, the injured area is far more susceptible to further injury.

Rehabilitation depends on an accurate diagnosis and specialist treatment and advice from doctors, physiotherapists, surgeons and strength and conditioning coaches for long-term success. There are three recognised stages of rehabilitation:

1 Early stage: gentle exercise encouraging damaged tissue to heal.
2 Mid stage: progressive loading of connective tissues and bones to develop strength.
3 Late stage: functional exercises and drills to ensure the body is ready to return to training.

Key term

Rehabilitation: the process of restoring full physical function after an injury has occurred.

55

Treatment methods

Stretching

The use of correct stretching techniques to rehabilitate injury can increase the speed of recovery. Using the wrong techniques at the wrong time could lead to further injury and delayed recovery:

- Acute phase: within the first three days of an injury no stretching should occur. PRICE and complete rest should be the focus. Stretching will cause more damage to the injured tissue.
- Mid phase: after three days, inflammation, bleeding and swelling should have subsided and gentle but active rehabilitation can start. For up to two weeks, heat therapy and gentle static and passive stretching exercises have proven to speed up the recovery process. The joint's connective tissues will be lightly moved into a slightly stretched position to increase the tension and allow tissues to lengthen. There should be no bouncing, jerky or forceful movements.
  - Research has shown four daily sessions of static stretching lead to shorter hamstring rehabilitation.
- Later phase: for a further two weeks range of motion, strength and co-ordination are focused on. PNF (proprioceptive neuromuscular facilitation) stretches are added to the continued static and passive stretching techniques. This will retrain and desensitise the stretch reflex, increase the range of motion, decrease sensations of pain and strengthen connective tissues.
- Long term: it is important to increase the range of motion and strength of connective tissues to a greater degree than when the injury occurred. Active and dynamic stretching through a developmental stretching programme should be used.

Study hint

Remember:
- Static stretching involves lengthening a muscle and connective tissue just beyond the point of resistance and holding for 10–30 seconds.
- Passive stretching involves assistance by a partner or piece of equipment to move a joint just beyond the point of resistance.
- PNF involves a static passive stretch, an isometric contraction of the agonist followed by relaxation and further stretch.
- Active stretching involves moving a joint into a stretched position with no assistance by contracting and strengthening the agonist muscle.
- Dynamic stretching involves moving a joint through its full range of motion with control over the entry and exit of the stretch, such as a walking lunge.
- Developmental stretching sessions are designed to improve the range of motion about a joint.

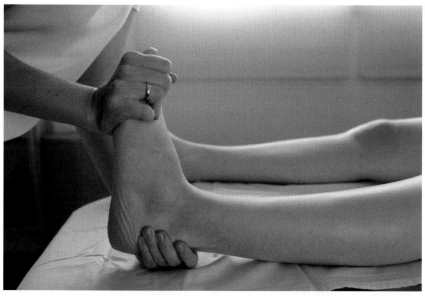

▲ Figure 2.1.22 Physiotherapist passively stretching the ankle joint

RESEARCH IN FOCUS

Page in 2012 published a summary of stretching research in the *International Journal of Sports Physical Therapy* titled 'Current concepts in muscle stretching for exercise and rehabilitation'. Based on the research, he recommended stretching was effective to increase muscle length, range of motion and collagen fibre alignment during rehabilitation of a healing muscle. PNF was most effective, with static stretching also beneficial, over a 6–8-week period to relieve tight hamstrings. Intensive static stretching was more effective than dynamic stretching for those recovering from hamstring strain. Static stretching was effective to increase range of motion about the knee joint for those with osteoarthritis, and post surgery (knee replacement) static, dynamic and PNF stretching was effective to increase range of motion. Researchers also show stretching programmes to be effective in reducing chronic pain by up to 94 per cent.

Extend your knowledge

Research post-isometric exercise relaxation (PIR) techniques as a gentle approach to increasing range of motion and relaxation, especially in the postural muscles associated with chronic pain. What are the differences from and similarities to PNF stretching?

Massage

Sports massage is a deep muscle therapy, realigning connective tissue fibres and flushing toxins from a damaged area. **Massage therapy** is a popular treatment for soft tissue injuries as well as part of an injury prevention programme by increasing joint mobility and flexibility. Depending on the specific injury and area of the body, sports massage can:

- move fluid and nutrients through damaged tissue to encourage healing and accelerate the removal of waste products
- stretch tissues, releasing tension and pressure and improving elasticity

Key term

Massage therapy: a physical therapy used for injury prevention and soft tissue injury treatment.

- break down scar tissue from previous injuries that can lead to inflexible tissues, injury and pain
- reduce pain and generate heat, circulation and relaxation.

Massage cannot be used on certain soft tissue injuries such as ligament or tendon ruptures (complete tear), contusions or open wounds as bleeding will be increased and the injury may be complicated.

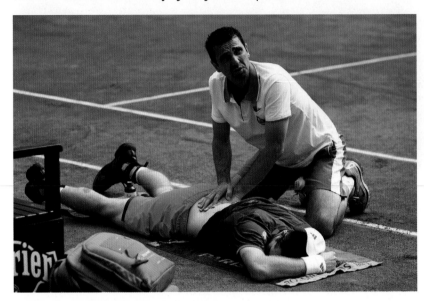

▲ Figure 2.1.23 Andy Murray receiving massage treatment on the side lines

Cold, heat and contrast therapies

The use of heat and cold is well researched and used by athletes and coaches post exercise to treat injuries and pain and boost recovery rates. The choice of cold, heat or contrast depends on the severity, type and nature of injury or damage.

Cold therapy is the use of ice or cold water to reduce tissue temperature, metabolic rate and speed of nerve impulses. It will also vasoconstrict blood vessels, decreasing blood flow, inflammation, swelling and pain associated with injury. Also known as cryotherapy, it is mainly used after acute injury for periods up to 20 minutes and reapplied every 1–3 hours.

- PRICE, applied as early as possible and continued for 24–48 hours, is the best treatment for acute soft tissue injuries. Ice packs are preferable to cold water immersion to maintain the effects of gravity.
- Cold water immersion (ice bath) for ten minutes at around 10°C has been shown to reduce the pain and drop in performance associated with exercise-induced muscle damage post exercise.
- Cryokinetics involves ice application followed by rehabilitation exercises, proven successful in treating ligament sprains.
- Cryostretching combines cold application and stretching to reduce muscle tension and increase flexibility, useful to decrease the pain associated with exercise-induced muscle damage.

Key terms

Cold therapy or cryotherapy: applying ice or cold to an injury or after exercise for a therapeutic effect, such as reduced swelling.
Heat therapy: applying heat to an area before training for a therapeutic effect, such as increased blood flow.
Contrast therapy: the use of alternate cold and heat for a therapeutic effect, such as increased blood flow.

Heat therapy is the use of heat to reduce muscle tension, stiffness and pain. It also vasodilates blood vessels, increasing blood flow and the healing response to a damaged area. Heat therapy is mainly used on chronic injuries and late-stage acute injuries around 48 hours post injury and during rehabilitation. It can also be used before exercise to raise the temperature of superficial muscles.

Heat therapy may include the use of heat packs, hot towels, heat rubs and warm water immersion for up to 20 minutes at a time. It may be combined with stretching to increase connective tissue elasticity during rehabilitation and before exercise. However, heat therapy should not be used in the acute phase of an injury as the greater blood flow will increase swelling.

Contrast therapy is the use of alternate cold and heat therapy to increase blood flow and decrease swelling and pain after exercise or in the late stage of injury. Once bleeding has stopped and inflammation has disappeared after the acute phase of an injury (3–5 days), contrast therapy can be used. The most common approach to contrast therapy is:

- to immerse the body up to shoulder level post exercise
- to use cold water followed immediately by warm water
- to have a cold:warm ratio of 1:3 or 1:4 minutes
- to have an accumulating 6–10 minutes in the cold water.

Applying cold vasoconstricts blood vessels and when followed immediately by heat, blood vessels vasodilate, causing a pumping action with large increases in blood flow and nutrient delivery for the damaged tissues. Research has shown contrast therapy to also reduce swelling and pain several days after injury and to be more effective than heat therapy alone to relieve the symptoms of exercise-induced muscle damage.

▼ Table 2.1.2 The benefits, risks and uses of heat, cold and contrast therapy

Therapy	Benefits	Risks	Uses
Heat	Vasodilation of blood vessels increasing blood flow, decreasing muscle tension, stiffness and pain	Increased swelling and pain after acute injury	Chronic injuries and late-stage acute injuries before exercise
Cold	Vasoconstriction of blood vessels decreasing blood flow, swelling and pain	Tissue and nerve damage if in contact for too long. Skin abrasions if direct contact (ice and skin)	Acute injuries and after exercise to relieve symptoms of exercise-induced muscle damage
Contrast	Large increases in blood flow and nutrient delivery to damaged tissue. Decreased swelling and pain	Limited benefit over and above cold therapy	Acute injuries after bleeding and inflammation have stopped and to relieve symptoms of exercise-induced muscle damage

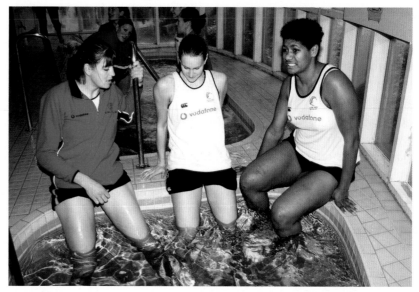

▲ Figure 2.1.24 The warm and cold water pools at the Australian Institute for Sport

Activity

Using the internet, search for the cold, heat and contrast therapies available at the Australian Institute for Sport and watch videos of recovery physiologist Dr Nathan Versey explaining their use and benefits to the elite athlete.

Anti-inflammatory drugs

Non-steroid anti-inflammatory drugs (NSAIDs), such as ibuprofen and aspirin, are commonly used in the treatment of acute sports injuries. Following an acute soft tissue injury, chemicals released by damaged cells cause vasodilation of blood vessels and an increase in blood and cellular fluid, which causes swelling and redness and activates pain receptors. Over-the-counter NSAIDs reduce this inflammatory response following tissue and cell damage by inhibiting the chemical release that leads to inflammation, interfering with pain signals and reducing temperature.

By using NSAIDs an athlete would aim to speed up the healing response and recovery time; however, they should do so with caution. Following acute injuries they may experience side effects of heartburn, nausea, headaches and diarrhoea. The inflammatory, painful first phase of the healing process should serve to prevent the athlete from doing further damage to the injured area by returning to training too early. The long-term use of NSAIDs in response to chronic injuries should be monitored by a heath professional as they can have significant health consequences, such as gastro-intestinal bleeding, shock, anaemia, stroke and heart attack.

Key term

Non-steroid anti-inflammatory drugs (NSAIDs): medication taken to reduce inflammation, temperature and pain following injury.

Physiotherapy

Physiotherapy is the treatment of injury or disease by qualified physiotherapists using physical methods. Physiotherapy treatment of musculoskeletal injuries, rather than drugs or surgery, may consist of:

- mobilisation and manipulation of joints and tissues
- electrotherapy to repair and stimulate tissues
- exercise therapy to strengthen muscles
- massage to stretch and relax tissues, relieve pain and increase circulation
- sport-specific rehabilitation programme design and advice
- posture and alignment training to release tension, minimise injury and maximise power output.

Key term

Physiotherapy: physical treatment of injuries and disease using methods such as mobilisation, massage, exercise therapy and postural training.

A dislocated shoulder during a rugby match, for example, will be diagnosed by a physiotherapist looking for signs of instability. Physiotherapy is then essential for recovery and an individualist programme should be followed, such as:

1 First phase: pain relief, minimise swelling, ice therapy and shoulder sling for support.

2 Second phase: tailored exercises to maintain rotator cuff muscle strength.

3 Third phase: restore normal range of motion, muscle length, connective tissue mobility and resting muscle tension about the shoulder joint with mobilisation, massage, stretching and possibly acupuncture.

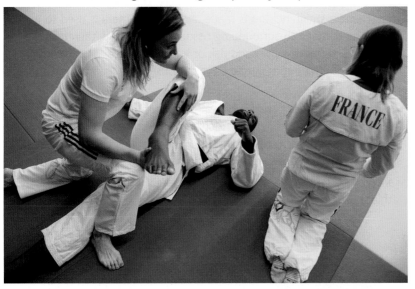

▲ Figure 2.1.25 Teddy Riner having physiotherapy treatment during a training session

Activity

Log on to the Chartered Society of Physiotherapy website and explore the different roles a physiotherapist undertakes and areas they can work in.

Extend your knowledge

Physiotherapists tend to work within four broad areas:
● neurological (for example, stroke, multiple sclerosis and Parkinson's patients)
● neuromusculoskeletal (for example, sports injuries, back pain and arthritis patients)
● cardiovascular (for example, heart disease and heart attack patients)
● respiratory (for example, asthma, cystic fibrosis and chronic obstructive pulmonary disorder patients).

They may work privately or within the NHS, research, education or management fields.

Surgery

Surgery is a relatively common procedure for elite sports athletes following serious injury or to combat persistent symptoms other treatments have failed to prevent. Sports injury-related surgical procedures include the repair of damaged soft tissue, realignment of bones and repositioning of joints:

● Knee ligament surgery. For example, anterior cruciate ligament (ACL) reconstruction in which, following rupture, a tissue graft (usually from the patella tendon) is used to replace the ACL and restore full function. Common for skiers.

- Shoulder stabilisation surgery. Following repeated dislocations surgery can be used to stabilise the shoulder joint by anchoring the humerus into the scapula and repairing the joint capsule, known as the Bankart repair. Common for throwing athletes.
- Meniscal tear surgery. Following cartilage tear in the knee surgical techniques aim to repair as much of the damaged cartilage as possible. Meniscus can be resurfaced to remove rough projections and in extreme cases a cartilage implant can be inserted. Common for footballers.

There are two main categories of surgical procedure depending on the severity and complexity of injury:

1   **Arthroscopy,** also known as keyhole surgery. Under general or local anaesthetic a small incision is made and a tiny camera is used to guide repair. The damage to surrounding tissues is minimised, therefore the athlete will suffer less pain and risk of infection and a faster initial recovery time than open surgery. Typically used to repair cartilage and soft tissue damage.

2   Open surgery. Under general or local anaesthetic an incision is made to open a joint to repair or reconstruct damaged structures. Although this can create a stronger repair, the risk of infection is high and scarring is significant. Typically used to repair fractures and reconstruct ankles.

Typical recovery times post surgery range from six weeks to several months. The athlete usually receives physiotherapy.

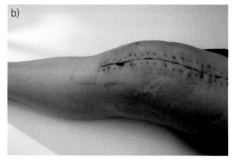

▲ Figure 2.1.26 Knee surgery: a) arthroscopy scars and b) open surgery scar

Treatment of common injuries

Fractures

Simple fractures are common in the sports arena: metatarsal bones (foot) in football, phalanges (fingers) in netball and the clavicle (collarbone) in rugby. The treatment will depend on the site and severity of the fracture, but medical attention will be required to assess the injury and immobilise the area correctly to encourage the healing process.

▼ Table 2.1.3 Signs, symptoms, potential causes and treatment of a simple fracture in sport

Simple fracture	Signs and symptoms	Potential causes
Break in a bone which causes little movement to the bone placement, minimising damage to the tissues	Severe pain at fracture site Loss of movement Swelling Discoloration	Excessive impact force from collision, falling or poor technique

Treatment
Depending on the site and severity of the simple fracture: ● medical attention and in severe cases an ambulance will be required ● PRICE to reduce swelling if it doesn't cause pain ● immobilisation using a splint, sling, crutches or plaster cast to assist the healing process ● anti-inflammatory and pain medication ● more severe fractures may require surgery to realign bones with the assistance of pins, wires or nails to fix the bones into their original position. Healing may take several weeks for a young performer, after a partial simple fracture of a finger, for example, to several months for an older performer after a more severe fracture. Physiotherapy will strengthen the connective tissues around the injured area and improve flexibility and mobility.

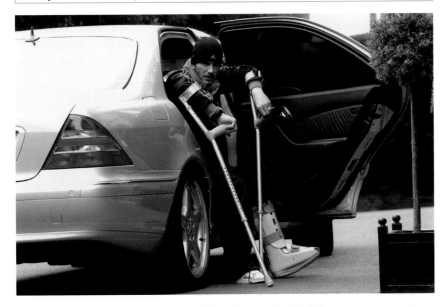

▲ Figure 2.1.27 David Beckham's immobilised foot and ankle following a metatarsal fracture

Stress fractures are common overuse injuries during training and performance, typically in the lower limb: tarsals, ankle, tibia and fibular bones of runners, tennis players, gymnasts and basketball players. The treatment will depend on the individual's ability to rest and totally avoid the activity or motion that caused the stress fracture for up to two months.

Stress fracture	Signs and symptoms	Potential causes
Tiny crack in the bone surface	Specific spots of pain during activity increasing with further use	Overtraining, intensity overload, fatigue, unfamiliar surfaces and inappropriate equipment use
Treatment		
In most cases: ● medical attention will be required for diagnosis and advice ● PRICE to reduce swelling ● rest for around two weeks and activity avoidance for a further eight to prevent larger, more complex stress fractures ● immobilisation may be used to limit activity using a splint or brace ● a gentle return to exercise accompanied by posture and alignment retraining ● strengthening exercises for surrounding connective tissue. Healing may take a significant period of time and, if rushed, a secondary, potentially worse injury may occur.		

Joint injuries

Dislocations can be common on the sports field, especially in contact or high-impact sports, such as a dislocated shoulder in rugby or hockey and a dislocated knee or ankle in dance or football. The treatment will depend on the site and severity of the dislocation, but medical attention will be required to assess the injury, immobilise the area and realign the joint correctly to encourage the healing process. Repeated dislocations of the same joint may lead to surgery and potentially the end of a sporting career.

▼ Table 2.1.5 Signs, symptoms, potential causes and treatment of a dislocation in sport

Dislocation	Signs and symptoms	Potential causes
Displacement of one bone from another from their original position	Severe pain, loss of movement, deformity, swelling and a 'pop' feeling	Excessive impact force from collision or fall
Treatment		
Depending on the site and severity of the dislocation: ● immediate medical attention, and in severe cases an ambulance will be required ● immobilisation using a splint or sling and no attempt to reposition bones unless by a medical professional ● PRICE to reduce swelling and relieve pain ● anti-inflammatory and pain medication ● more severe or repeated dislocations may require surgery to realign and pin bones into their original position. Physiotherapy will strengthen the connective tissues around the joint and improve flexibility and mobility.		

Sprain injuries are common in dynamic sports with changes of direction and twisting actions, such as ankle sprains in netball, basketball and football players and knee sprains in skiers. The treatment will depend on the site and severity of the sprain from first (overstretch) to third degree (detachment).

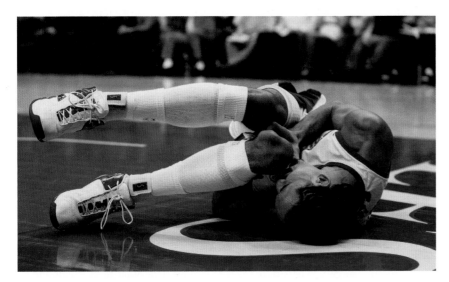

▲ Figure 2.1.28 Basketball player Shaun Livingston ruptured cruciate ligaments and dislocated his patella and tibia from the knee joint after a bad landing from a lay-up shot

▼ Table 2.1.6 Signs, symptoms, potential causes and treatment of a sprain in sport

Sprain	Signs and symptoms	Potential causes
Damage to the ligaments that connect bone to bone (overstretch, rupture or detachment)	Pain, swelling, discoloration and inability to bear weight	Sudden twist, impact or fall that forces the joint beyond its extreme range of motion

Treatment
Depending on the site and severity of the sprain: ● medical attention may be required in severe cases (second- and third-degree sprains) ● PRICE to reduce swelling ● immobilisation or support using strapping, a brace or crutches to assist the healing process ● anti-inflammatory and pain medication ● functional rehabilitation, strengthening, mobility and balance exercises ● third-degree severe sprains in rare cases may require reconstructive surgery. Recovery can take from several weeks to several months and surgery will take place only as the result of a failure to respond to non-surgical treatments.

A torn cartilage is a common joint injury in sport which can affect the articular cartilage in the shoulder, elbow or hip, but is largely associated with fibrocartilage in the knee joint. At the top of the tibia lie two discs of fibrocartilage called **menisci**, which stabilise the knee joint and act as shock absorbers during weight-bearing activity. A sudden twist as the joint is bearing weight can cause the menisci to get jammed between the two bones and if there is excessive force a tear may occur. A torn cartilage injury may be seen in athletes performing dynamic, twisting, pivoting, cutting or decelerating activities, such as football, and should receive immediate PRICE treatment. Medical attention will be necessary and persistent cases will often require surgery.

Key term

Menisci: a tough disc of fibrocartilage in the knee joint which stabilises and absorbs shock during weight-bearing activity.

▼ Table 2.1.7 Signs, symptoms, potential causes and treatment of a torn cartilage

Torn cartilage	Signs and symptoms	Potential causes
A tear in the articular or fibrocartilage within a joint, such as the meniscus of the knee	Associated damage to the ligaments which causes pain and swelling. A 'clunking' or 'popping' sensation and locking of the knee	Sudden twist, impact or fall, torn ligaments and dislocation

Treatment
Depending on the site and severity of the tear: • medical attention will be required • PRICE to reduce pain and swelling • anti-inflammatory and pain medication • physiotherapy to strengthen connective tissues and restore range of motion • knee brace to aid joint stability can be worn • hydrotherapy (exercises in the water) to maintain fitness without bearing weight • arthroscopy surgery in persistent cases to remove flaps or jagged sections and to smooth the meniscus (resurfacing). Cartilage does not have a blood supply and so recovery can be slow. Athletes can typically start participating in their sport two months post surgery.

IN THE NEWS

In preparation for the 2014 football World Cup Uruguay striker Luis Suarez damaged the meniscus in his left knee during training. He underwent arthroscopy surgery shortly afterwards and to the surprise of many, returned to the playing field within four weeks. Doctors agree Suarez's fitness levels would have helped his recovery, and physiotherapy and strength conditioning would have played a large role in rehabilitation. A football manager would be delighted; however, orthopaedic surgeons might worry at the speedy return to match play, with potential risks of more serious knee problems such as arthritis in the future. Suarez was stretchered off visibly tired and in pain before the end of his return match where Uruguay beat England 2–1.

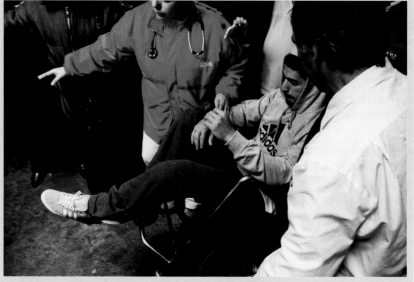

▲ Figure 2.1.29 Footballer Luis Suarez post meniscus surgery

Exercise-induced muscle damage

Exercise-induced muscle damage is a familiar experience for athletes, common at the beginning of a training programme, new activity or after a period of rest. Eccentric exercise such as strength training, downhill running and plyometrics causes microscopic injury to the muscle fibres. The greater the intensity and duration of eccentric exercise, the greater the exercise-induced muscle damage. Symptoms include pain, tenderness, swelling, stiffness and a decreased range of motion and strength peaking 24–72 hours post exercise, hence its common reference as 'delayed onset muscle soreness'. A warm up, stretching routine and gradual increases in intensity and duration will lessen the impact of exercise-induced muscle damage. Treatment using cold therapy, massage or medication will reduce the associated pain.

▼ Table 2.1.8 Signs, symptoms, potential causes and treatment of exercise-induced muscle damage in sport

Exercise-induced muscle damage	Signs and symptoms	Potential causes
Microscopic injury to the muscle fibres	Pain, tenderness, swelling, stiffness, decreased range of motion and strength peaking 24–72 hours post exercise	Excessive eccentric exercise

Treatment
In most cases medical attention is not required and symptoms should stop within five days. Research has shown methods to treat the muscle damage itself to be ineffective; however, the pain associated with DOMS can be reduced by: ● cold therapy such as ice pack application or ice bath post exercise ● massage and stretching techniques ● anti-inflammatory and pain medication. Medical attention should be sought if there is heavy swelling or dark urine as this may indicate the level of muscle damage has affected the kidneys.

Summary

Injuries in sport are common and range from minor scrapes to serious medical emergencies. Injury prevention and rehabilitation is essential to a long playing career and active, healthy lifestyle.

- Acute injuries are sudden and associated with a traumatic event, such as a sprained ankle in cross country running or concussion in rugby. Chronic injuries occur over a period of time and are associated with repeated or continuous stress, such as tennis elbow.
- Hard tissue injuries are damage to the bone, joint or cartilage, such as:
  - Fractures: a partial or complete break in a bone due to excessive force.
  - Dislocations: the displacement of bones from their original position.
  - Stress fracture: a tiny crack in the surface of a bone caused by overuse.
- Soft tissue injuries are damage to the connective tissues, such as:
  - Strains and sprains: overstretch or torn muscles, tendons or ligaments.
  - Shin splints: chronic shin pain due to inflammation of muscles and tendon attachments to the tibia.
  - Tendinosis: deterioration of a tendon due to overuse.
- Intrinsic injury risk factors come from within the body and include individual variables, such as previous injury, and training effects, such as poor preparation. Extrinsic injury risk factors come from outside the body and include poor technique, incorrect equipment and inappropriate overload in training.

Study hint

It is a common misunderstanding to think exercise-induced muscle damage is caused by lactic acid accumulation. Lactic acid accumulation causes acute onset muscle soreness during an activity, not the delayed onset muscle soreness associated with muscle damage.

Evaluation

Common treatments:
- PRICE to reduce swelling and pain.
- Immobilisation to protect unstable limbs or joints.
- Anti-inflammatory and pain medication to reduce swelling and pain.
- Rest to prevent further damage and allow the body's natural healing response.
- Physiotherapy to rehabilitate and restore function (strength, stability and mobility).
- Surgery to repair severe damage such as complete tears or fractures.

Activity

Summarise sports injuries and rehabilitation by creating a table, poster or spider diagram split into two sections: acute and chronic injuries. Define and give examples of hard and soft tissues, and state potential causes and treatment methods.

Check your understanding

1 Answer the following statements as true or false:
 a Chronic injuries are often referred to as overuse injuries.
 b A strain is an overstretch or tear in a bone-to-bone connecting ligament.
 c A stress fracture is a tiny crack in the surface of a bone caused by an acute impact.
 d The six Rs to recognise concussion are: recognise, remove, refer, rest, recover and return.
 e Arthroscopy is a surgical procedure to examine and repair damage within a joint.
 f Cold therapy is the use of ice or cold water to treat injury and reduce inflammation before exercise.
 g A warm up should contain dynamic stretches and a cool down should contain static stretches.
 h An anti-inflammatory drug, such as ibuprofen, can be taken to reduce inflammation, temperature and pain following an injury.

2 Identify the key terms from the following statements:
 a Type of injury to the bone, joint or cartilage, such as a fracture or dislocation.
 b A traumatic brain injury resulting in a loss of brain function, such as dizziness.
 c Tendon pain in the forearm due to repetitive strain and chronic overuse associated with racket sports.
 d The process of restoring full physical function after an injury.
 e Physical therapy using techniques such as mobilisation, massage and postural training.

Practice questions

1 Define and give an example of acute and chronic injuries to the soft tissues. (4 marks)
2 Describe the PRICE protocol for the immediate treatment of acute injuries. (5 marks)
3 Describe and explain the benefits of sports massage. (4 marks)
4 Using a sport of your choice, describe an appropriate warm up routine and explain its benefits with reference to the skeletal, muscular and cardiovascular systems. Discuss the risk factors for injury and how they can be controlled in your sport. (20 marks)

Part 3
Biomechanics

3.1 Linear motion

Understanding the specification

By the end of this chapter you should be able to demonstrate knowledge and understanding of linear motion, and how it is created and measured in the performance of physical activities and sport:

- characteristics and creation of linear motion
- key descriptors: distance, displacement, speed, velocity, acceleration and deceleration
- distance/time, speed/time and velocity/time graphs of linear motion.

Key terms

Linear motion: movement of a body in a straight or curved line, where all parts move the same distance, in the same direction over the same time.

Direct force: a force applied through the centre of mass resulting in linear motion.

Centre of mass: the point at which a body is balanced in all directions. The point from which weight appears to act.

Linear motion

Biomechanics is the study of human movement and the effect of force and motion on sport performance. Depending on where a force is applied to a body, differing forms of motion can be created.

Linear motion is movement of a body in a straight or curved line, where all parts move the same distance, in the same direction over the same time. For example, a water skier on a flat lake being pulled at constant speed will travel in linear motion as all parts of their body will travel in the same direction over the same distance per unit of time. Equally, a bob skeleton rider hitting the final straight at top speed will have all their body parts travelling in the same direction, over the same distance per unit of time.

Linear motion results from a **direct force** being applied to a body, where the force is applied directly to the **centre of a body's mass** (or centre force).

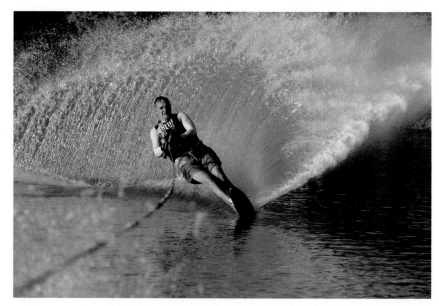

▲ Figure 3.1.1 A water skier travelling in linear motion as his body travels in a straight or curved line at constant speed

According to Newton's first law of motion, an uninterrupted body will continue to travel in linear motion indefinitely. In a sporting context this is rarely the case due to the forces previously studied, such as air resistance, which will act on a body to cause deceleration.

Linear motion descriptors

Being able to describe motion is essential to analyse performance. With the correct descriptors, calculations can be made assessing speed, velocity and acceleration over the whole and different parts of an event, such as the sprint start of a 100 m or final 400 m of a 5,000 m. These data can be used to analyse performance and identify strengths and weaknesses.

There are five key descriptors important in this section, which can be calculated to build data and create a picture of performance:

1 Distance.
2 Displacement.
3 Speed.
4 Velocity.
5 Acceleration/deceleration.

Distance

Distance is the total length of the path covered from start to finish (or position A to B). Distance is measured in metres (m), for example:

- The distance covered in the 100 m sprint is 100 m, swimming four lengths of a 50 m pool is 200 m (4 × 50 m) and the London marathon from start to finish is 42,195 m.

Displacement

Displacement is the shortest straight-line route from start to finish (or position A to B). Displacement is measured in metres (m), for example:

- The displacement covered in the 100 m sprint is 100 m, swimming four lengths of a 50 m pool is 0 m and the London marathon is around 10,000 m.

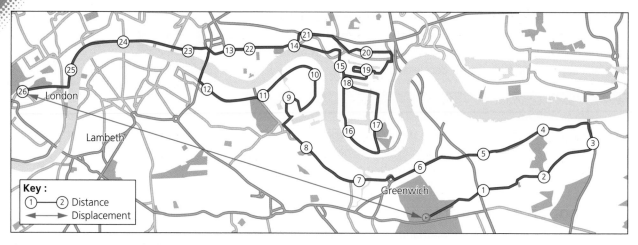

▲ Figure 3.1.2 Distance vs displacement in the London marathon

Speed

Speed is the rate of change in distance and can be calculated using the following equation:

$$\text{Speed} = \text{distance} / \text{time taken}$$

Speed is measured in metres per second (m/s), distance in metres (m) and time taken in seconds (s), for example:

- Dafne Schippers broke the 200 m record with a time of 21.63 s. The distance from the start to the finish line is 200 m. The average speed over the whole race is 9.25 m/s (average speed = 200 m/21.63 s).

Velocity

Velocity is the rate of change in displacement and can be calculated using the following equation:

$$\text{Velocity} = \text{displacement} / \text{time taken}$$

Velocity is measured in metres per second (m/s), displacement in metres (m) and time taken in seconds (s), for example:

- Usain Bolt broke the world 100 m sprint record in 2009 with a time of 9.58 s. The displacement from the start to the finish line is 100 m. The average velocity over the whole race is 10.44 m/s (average velocity = 100 m/9.58 s).

Acceleration/deceleration

Acceleration is the rate of change in velocity and can be calculated using the following equation:

$$\text{Acceleration} = (\text{final velocity} - \text{initial velocity}) / \text{time taken}$$

Acceleration is measured in metres per second per second (m/s/s), change in velocity in metres per second (m/s) and time taken in seconds (s), for example:

- When Usain Bolt ran the 100 m in 9.58 s (Berlin, 2009), his split time over the first 20 m was 2.89 s. His velocity at 20 m was 6.92 m/s (20 m/ 2.89 s) and his velocity at 0 m was 0.00 m/s (0 m/0.00 s).

- The change in velocity is 6.92 m/s (6.92 − 0.00) and when divided by the split time (2.89 s) his average acceleration out of the blocks and over the first 20 m is 2.39 m/s/s.

Deceleration occurs when the rate of change in velocity is negative or there is a decrease in velocity over time, for example:

- As a sprinter crosses the finish line they will lean back and push down against the track to decelerate. As they cross the finish line they may be travelling around 9 m/s, two seconds later they may be travelling at 5 m/s. The sprinter is therefore decelerating at a rate of 2 m/s/s (final velocity − initial velocity / time taken, 5 − 9 m/s / 2s).
- In the same way a freestyle swimmer will push off the race blocks accelerating towards the water; however, as they enter the water the

Study hint

When posed with an exam question on acceleration, remember the equation to calculate force can also be rearranged:

Force = mass × acceleration

Acceleration = force / mass

The units will remain the same (m/s/s). If the result is positive, acceleration is occurring; if the result is negative, deceleration is occurring; and if the result is zero, there is no acceleration and the body is either at rest or travelling with constant velocity.

IN THE NEWS

2015 Formula 1 British Grand Prix winner Lewis Hamilton drove to victory with the fastest lap time of 97.1 s. One lap of the circuit at Silverstone is 5,891 m in distance; therefore, Hamilton's top average speed around the track was 60.67 m/s. The Mercedes F1 W06 Hybrid has an estimated top speed of around 321.87 km per hour (200 mph) and can accelerate from 0–60 m in just three seconds. The F1 car is all important to the success of the driver, as Hamilton found with his disappointing performances in early years in cars such as the McLaren MP4-25, when he was outpaced by rivals Red Bull and Ferrari.

Study hint

Distance and speed are measures of size only, whereas displacement, velocity and acceleration are measures of size and direction, giving a more precise picture of motion.

Activity

Use the following data from the 2015 IAAF World Championships men's events to compare the average speed attained in the various athletic track events:

Distance (m)	Time taken (s)	Competitor	Average speed (m/s)
100	9.79	Usain Bolt	
200	19.55	Usain Bolt	
400	43.48	Wayde van Niekerk	
800	105.84	David Rudisha	
1,500	214.40	Asbel Kiprop	
5,000	830.38	Mohamed Farah	
10,000	1,621.13	Mohamed Farah	

Evaluation

Distance: the total length covered from start to finish (m).
Displacement: shortest straight-line route from start to finish (m).
Speed: distance/time taken (m/s).
Velocity: displacement/time taken (m/s).
Acceleration: (final velocity − initial velocity) / time taken (m/s/s).

Graphs of linear motion

Graphs of linear motion can be used to represent the motion of a body moving in a straight or curved path. The key descriptors of linear motion can be recorded and plotted using three graphs:

a Distance/time.

b Speed/time.

c Velocity/time.

These graphs can be used to gain a quick visual representation of complex data, identify patterns of motion, and calculate speed or acceleration at a particular moment in time.

Distance/time graphs

A **distance/time graph** shows the distance a body travels over a period of time. The **gradient** of the curve indicates the speed of the body at a particular instant and will show whether the body is at rest, travelling with constant speed, accelerating or decelerating. Using the distance/time curve, speed can be calculated at any given point using the formula:

Speed = distance/time

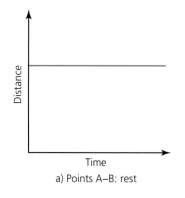

a) Points A–B: rest

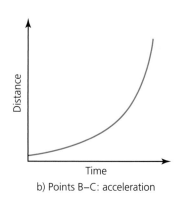

b) Points B–C: acceleration

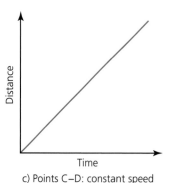

c) Points C–D: constant speed

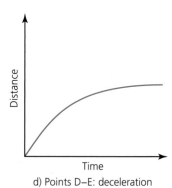

d) Points D–E: deceleration

▲ Figure 3.1.3 Stages of motion represented with distance/time graphs, a) rest, b) acceleration, c) constant speed and d) deceleration

The distance/time graph in Figure 3.1.4 shows each type of motion, between:

- Points A–B: the horizontal line shows time increasing but no change in distance. This represents a rest or a stationary position. The sprinter is at rest in the blocks.
- Points B–C: the increasing gradient (positive curve) shows distance increasing per unit of time. This represents an increasing rate of speed or acceleration. The sprinter drives out of the blocks and accelerates down the track.
- Points C–D: the straight diagonal line shows the same increase in distance per unit of time. This represents constant speed. The sprinter has reached maximum speed around 40 m and tries to maintain it for as long as possible.
- Points D–E: the decreasing gradient shows distance decreasing per unit of time. This represents a decreasing rate of speed or deceleration. The sprinter fatigues or crosses the finish line.

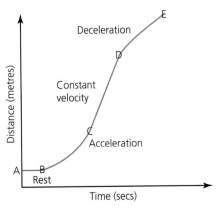

▲ Figure 3.1.4 A distance/time graph showing the motion of a 100 m sprinter

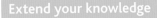
Extend your knowledge

The gradient of a graph at a particular moment in time can be calculated using the equation:

Gradient of graph = change in y axis / change in × axis

Speed/time graphs

A **speed/time graph** shows the speed of a body over a period of time. The gradient of the curve indicates the acceleration of the body at a particular instant and will show whether the body is at rest, travelling with constant speed, accelerating or decelerating. Using the speed/time curve, distance travelled can be measured as the area under the speed/time curve is equal to the distance travelled by a body.

Activity

Using Figure 3.1.4, apply Newton's laws of motion to specific sections of the race:

- Newton's first law to A–B and C–D
- Newton's second law to B–C and D–E
- Newton's third law to B.

Key term

Speed/time graph: a visual representation of the speed of motion plotted against the time taken.

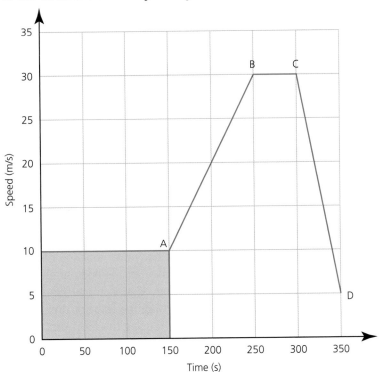

▲ Figure 3.1.5 A speed/time graph showing the distance travelled shaded in green

The speed/time graph in Figure 3.1.5 shows each type of motion, between:

- Points 0–A: the horizontal line shows a constant speed maintained as time increases. The shaded area underneath this section of the curve shows a distance covered of 1,500 m (10 m/s × 150 s).
- Points A–B: the increasing gradient (positive curve) shows speed increasing per unit of time from 10 m/s up to 30 m/s. This represents acceleration.
- Points B–C: the horizontal line again shows constant speed.
- Points C–D: the decreasing gradient shows speed decreasing per unit of time from 30 m/s back down to 10 m/s. This represents deceleration.

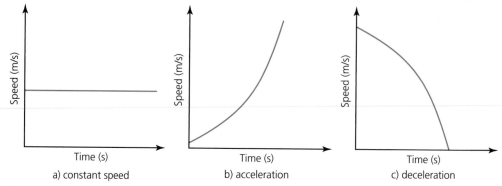

▲ Figure 3.1.6 Stages of motion represented with speed/time graphs, a) constant speed, b) acceleration and c) deceleration

Activity

Using Figure 3.1.7, answer the following questions:

1 At what speed is the sprinter travelling at four seconds?
2 Calculate the acceleration of the sprinter between two and four seconds.
3 Describe the motion of the 100 m sprinter from points A–B and B–C.

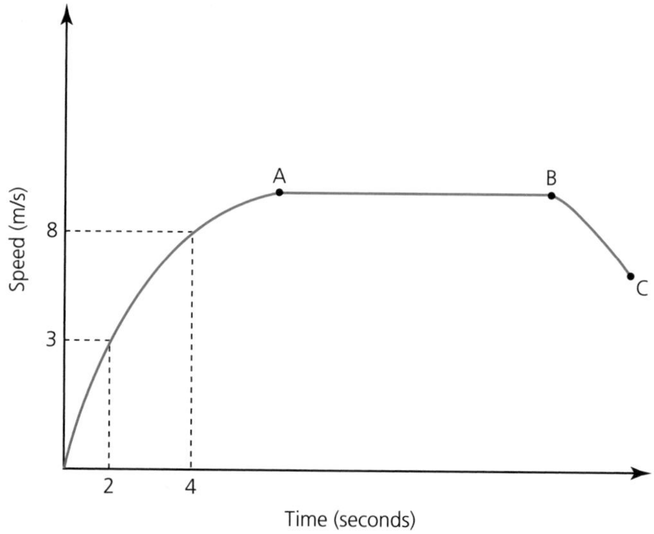

▲ Figure 3.1.7 A speed/time graph showing the motion of a 100 m sprinter completing a race

Key term

Velocity/time graph: a visual representation of the velocity of motion plotted against the time taken.

Velocity/time graphs

A **velocity/time graph** shows the velocity of a body over a period of time. The gradient of the curve indicates the acceleration of the body at a particular instant and will show whether the body is at rest, travelling with uniform velocity, accelerating or decelerating. Using the velocity/time curve, acceleration can be calculated at any given point using the formula:

Acceleration = (final velocity – initial velocity) / time

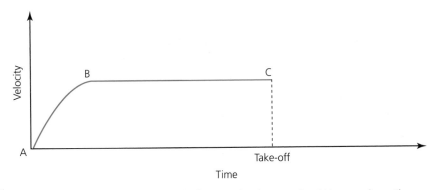

▲ Figure 3.1.8 A velocity/time graph showing the descent of a ski jumper down the ramp prior to take-off

The velocity/time graph in Figure 3.1.8 shows three types of motion:

- Point A: on the horizontal axis velocity = 0. This represents a rest or stationary position. The ski jumper is seated, ready to stand.
- Points A–B: the upward curve shows an increase in velocity per unit of time. This represents an increasing rate of velocity or acceleration. The ski jumper accelerates down the ramp.
- Points B–C: the horizontal line shows no change in velocity per unit of time. This represents uniform velocity. The ski jumper reaches uniform velocity, which is maintained until take-off.

A velocity/time graph can also show any change in direction the body makes. A negative curve below the horizontal axis represents a change in the body's direction.

The velocity/time graph shown in Figure 3.1.9 represents each type of motion, between:

- Points A–B: acceleration. Player A applied a force to accelerate the ball towards player B.
- Points B–C: deceleration (the downward curve shows a decrease in velocity per unit of time). Player B cushions the ball to decelerate it to a resting position at point C.
- Points C–D: rest. Player B controls the ball and prepares to return the pass.
- Points D–E: acceleration followed by deceleration in the opposite direction. Player B applies a force to the ball, accelerating it back to player A, who cushions the ball, decelerating it to rest.

Study hint

If you are finding it difficult to interpret a velocity/time graph, place numbers on the vertical axis, with positive numbers increasing upwards from 0 on the horizontal axis and negative numbers increasing downwards from 0 on the horizontal axis.

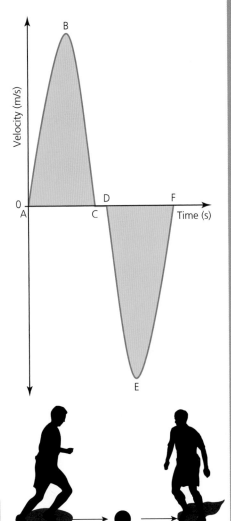

▲ Figure 3.1.9 A velocity/time graph showing the motion of a ball being passed between two players

a)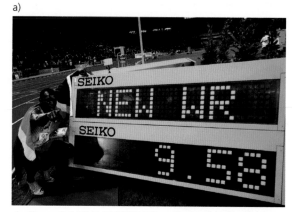

b)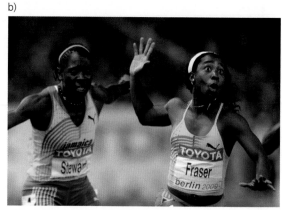

▲ Figure 3.1.10 IAAF 2009 100 m finals: a) Usain Bolt's world record of 9.58 s and b) Fraser-Pryce's 10.73 s win

Activity

Using the table below draw a distance/time graph to represent the motion of Usain Bolt and Shelly-Ann Fraser-Pryce over the 2009 IAAF World Championship 100 m races. Carefully plot the split times every 20 m against time on the horizontal axis and distance on the vertical axis. Using your graph, analyse the motion plotted and compare the two sprinters.

	0 m	20 m	40 m	60 m	80 m	100 m
Bolt	0.00 s	2.88 s	4.64 s	6.31 s	7.92 s	9.58 s
Fraser-Pryce	0.00 s	3.03 s	4.98 s	6.88 s	8.77 s	10.73 s

Using the graph you produce, answer the following questions:
1 Compare Bolt and Fraser-Pryce's average speed over the whole 100 m race.
2 Compare Bolt and Fraser-Pryce's speed at 50 m.
Calculate the velocity at each 20 m interval for both athletes and draw a velocity/time graph with your results. Using your graph, answer the following questions:
1 Compare the maximum velocity achieved by Bolt and Fraser-Pryce.
2 Compare Bolt and Fraser-Pryce's average acceleration over the first 10 m of the sprint.

Activity

If you have the facilities, select two members of the class and recreate a 100 m race with markers every 20 m. After a sufficient warm up and using a stopwatch, record the split times as each performer passes the 20 m markers. Add your classmates' results to the distance/time graph created and discuss any similarities and differences.
● Extend this activity and calculate the velocity each performer is running with at each 20 m interval. Draw a velocity/time graph with your results and note the motion of each performer at different times during the race. Identify any times of acceleration, constant velocity and deceleration.

RESEARCH IN FOCUS

Graubner, R. and Nixdorf, E. (2011) 'Biomechanical analysis of the sprint and hurdles events at the 2009 IAAF World Championships in Athletics', *Positions*, 1: 10.

This research paper provides a biomechanical analysis of elite sprinters and hurdlers. Video recordings and laser measurement systems were used to provide split times, stride length and stride frequency data on the men's and women's finals. Results are shown in table and graph format with accompanying photographs.

Activity

Using Graubner and Nixdorf's biomechanical analysis of the 200 m sprint at the 2009 IAAF World Championships, practise application of the knowledge and understanding you have gained so far. The discussion and presentation of data on the 200 m sprint begins on page 31 at www.meathathletics.ie/devathletes/pdf/Biomechanics%20of%20Sprints.pdf). See what you can do with the data, for example:

1 Using the split times, plot a distance/time graph and analyse the results of the men's final.
2 Using the mean velocities at 50 m intervals, plot a velocity/time graph and analyse the results of the men's final.
3 Compare Usain Bolt's performance in the 100 m and 200 m races.

Summary

Linear motion is a key concept in biomechanics and its descriptors are commonly used to analyse performance in physical activities:

- Linear motion is movement in a straight or curved line, where all parts move the same distance, in the same direction over the same time. It is a result of a direct force being applied to a body to create motion.
- The five key descriptors of linear motion are:
  - Distance: total length of the path covered from start to finish (m).
  - Displacement: shortest straight-line route from start to finish (m).
  - Speed: the rate of change in distance (m/s). Speed = distance/time taken.
  - Velocity: the rate of change in displacement (m/s). Velocity = displacement/time taken.
  - Acceleration: the rate of change in velocity (m/s/s). Acceleration = (final velocity – initial velocity) / time taken.
- Graphs are drawn to visually represent the motion of a body and provide the basis for calculations of speed (distance/time graph) or acceleration (speed/time and velocity/time graphs) to be made.

1 Answer the following statements as true or false:
   a A 100 m sprinter is a good example of linear motion.
   b Linear motion can result from movement in a straight and a curved path.
   c The distance covered when a 1,500 m runner completes their race is 0 m.
   d The displacement of a 50 m butterfly swimmer in a 50 m Olympic pool is 50 m.
   e Speed is calculated using the formula: speed = distance/time taken.
   f Velocity is measured in metres per second per second (m/s/s).
   g The slope of a graph at a particular moment in time is known as the gradient.
   h Acceleration can be calculated using a velocity/time graph.

2 Identify the key terms from the following statements:
   a A force applied through the centre of mass.
   b Movement of a body in a straight or curved line, where all parts move the same distance, in the same direction over the same time.
   c The shortest straight-line route from start to finish position.
   d The negative rate of change in velocity (m/s/s).
   e A visual representation of the distance travelled plotted against the time taken.

Practice questions

1 Explain how distance and displacement differ in the 200 m freestyle swimming event. (4 marks)

2 If a track cyclist completes a 1,000 m time trial in 58.87 s, what is their average speed during the race? (2 marks)

3 Sketch a velocity/time graph showing the motion of a tennis ball served from player A to player B and returned by player B to player A. Explain the shape of your velocity/time graph. (6 marks)

4 An athlete performs a 100 m sprint. They show four phases of motion:

   a They are stationary in the blocks.
   b They quickly move away from the blocks.
   c They achieve their fastest pace and maintain this for 30 m.
   d They begin to fatigue and slow down as they approach the finish line.

Sketch a distance/time graph to represent the sprinter's motion throughout the race and identify the type of motion shown in each phase.

Using Newton's laws of motion, analyse the sprint start out of the blocks. Finally, identify and describe the forces acting on the sprinter as they achieve and maintain their fastest pace during the race. (20 marks)

3.2 Angular motion

Understanding the specification

By the end of this chapter you should be able to demonstrate knowledge and understanding of angular motion, and how it is created, measured and conserved in the performance of physical activities and sport:

- characteristics and creation of angular motion
- axes of rotation
- key descriptors: moment of inertia, angular velocity and angular momentum
- graphs of moment of inertia, angular velocity and angular momentum
- conservation of angular momentum
- angular analogue of Newton's first law of motion.

Angular motion

Linear motion is rare in sport due to the dynamic nature of most physical activities and the effects of friction and air resistance acting on a body in motion. Objects tend to rotate as they pass over a surface – for example, the wheels of a F1 car or track bike. Projectiles tend to rotate as they pass through the air – for instance, a discus or tennis ball.

Angular motion is movement of a body or part of a body in a circular path about an axis of rotation. For example, a gymnast's whole body will rotate around the high bar (axis of rotation), an athlete's legs rotate at the hip joint (axis of rotation) as they run, and a trampolinist's whole body rotates around their centre of mass during a somersault.

> **Key term**
>
> **Angular motion:** movement of a body or part of a body in a circular path about an axis of rotation.

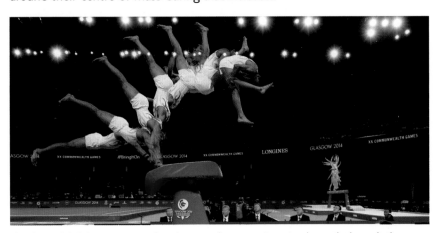

▲ Figure 3.2.1 A gymnast performing a vault rotates in a circular path through the air. The gymnast rotates around the hip, which acts as the axis of rotation

Angular motion results from an **eccentric force** being applied to a body, where the force is applied outside the centre of a body's mass. An eccentric force is also known as **torque** – a turning or rotational force. The understanding of angular motion is critical for performance analysis and technique perfection due to the skeletal make-up of the human body: bones act as levers which move about a joint (fulcrum) and create a form of rotational movement, such as flexion or abduction.

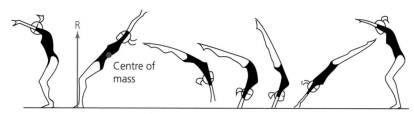

▲ Figure 3.2.2 A gymnast uses an eccentric force as the external force (reaction) passes outside the centre of mass at take-off to produce backward rotation

Table 3.2.1 A comparison of linear and angular motion

	Linear motion	**Angular motion**
Definition	Linear motion is movement of a body in a straight or curved line, where all parts move the same distance, in the same direction over the same time	Angular motion is movement of a body in a circular path about an axis of rotation
Created by	Direct force An external force passes through the centre of mass	Eccentric force An external force passes outside the centre of mass
Sporting example	Skeleton bob at top speed	Gymnastic somersault Drive and recovery leg rotating about the hip joint of a runner Arm rotating about the shoulder joint of a tennis player serving

Principal axes of rotation

If an eccentric force is applied to a body, it will rotate around one (or more) of three principal axes of rotation. A **principal axis of rotation** is an imaginary line that passes through the centre of mass about which a performer can rotate:

● Longitudinal axis runs from head to toe through the centre of mass. A body rotating around the longitudinal axis would be performing actions such as a flat spin on the ice or full turn in trampolining.

● Transverse axis runs from left to right through the centre of mass. A body rotating around the transverse axis would be performing actions such as somersaults.

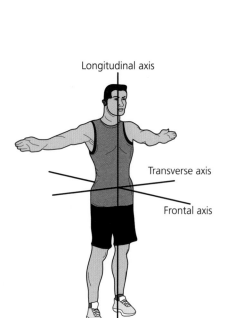

▲ Figure 3.2.3 The principal axes of rotation

- Frontal axis runs from front to back through the centre of mass. A body rotating around the frontal axis would be performing actions such as cartwheels.

a)
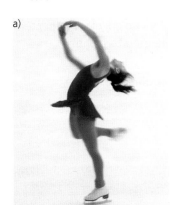

b)
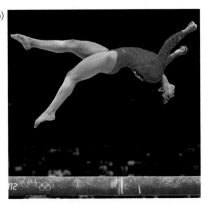

c)
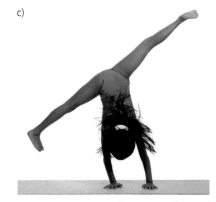

▲ Figure 3.2.4 Movement about the principal axes of rotation: a) longitudinal rotation: an ice skater performing a flat spin on the ice, b) transverse rotation: a gymnast performing a backward somersault on the beam, c) frontal rotation: a gymnast performing a cartwheel

Activity

Fill in the blanks in the following paragraph:

Angular motion is movement of a body or part of a body in a _____ path about an axis of _____. It is created by applying an _____ force to a body. This is where an external force passes _____ the centre of _____. A measure of the turning force applied to the body is known as _____. A body can rotate around three principal axes: the _____ axis of rotation (for example, a ballet dancer performing a pirouette), the _____ axis of rotation (for example, a swimmer performing a tumble turn) and the _____ axis of rotation (for example, a goalkeeper diving to the top corner to make a save).

Extend your knowledge

Movement at a joint takes place along a plane about an axis linking anatomy and physiology to biomechanics. Examples of movement around the dominant planes of motion and axes of rotation are:

- sagittal plane of motion (flexion and extension) about the frontal axis of rotation – for example, walking, squatting and overhead press
- frontal plane of motion (abduction, adduction and lateral flexion) about the transverse axis of rotation – for example, star jumps and side bends
- transverse plane of motion (rotation, supination and pronation) about the longitudinal axis of rotation – for example, throwing and golf swings.

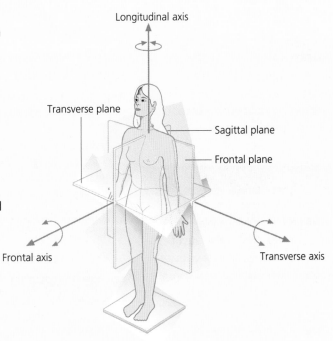

▲ Figure 3.2.5 The principal axes of rotation and planes of motion

Angular motion descriptors

Being able to describe angular motion is essential to analyse technical aspects of performance. With the correct descriptors calculations can be made assessing moment of inertia, angular velocity and angular momentum over different parts of an event. The results can be used to identify strengths and weaknesses.

The three key descriptors important to angular motion are:

1 Angular velocity.

2 Moment of inertia.

3 Angular momentum.

Key term

Radian (rad): a unit of measurement of the angle through which a body rotates. $360° = 2\pi$ radians, 1 radian = 57.3 degrees.

Study hint

Angular motion is measured in **radians**. A radian is a unit of measurement of the angle through which a body rotates. Angular distance and angular displacement are measured in radians, angular speed and angular velocity in radians per second (rad/s).

Extend your knowledge

Knowledge of angular descriptors is important to gain a full picture of an athlete's ability to rotate. In the same way as using descriptors of linear motion to analyse performance, angular distance, angular displacement, angular speed and angular acceleration can also be calculated:

- Angular distance is the total angle a body turns through from start to finish position when rotating about an axis (rad).
- Angular displacement is the smallest angle between the start and finish position of a body rotating about an axis (rad).
- Angular speed is the rate of change in angular distance (rad/s).
  - Angular speed = angular distance/time taken.
- Angular acceleration is the rate of change in angular velocity (rad/s/s).
  - Angular acceleration = (final – initial angular velocity)/time taken.

Key term

Angular velocity: the rate of change in angular displacement measured in radians per second (rate of spin).

Angular velocity

Angular velocity is the rate of change in angular displacement or simply the rate of rotation. It can be calculated using the following equation:

Angular velocity = angular displacement/time taken

Angular velocity is measured in radians per second (rad/s), angular displacement in radians (rad) and time taken in seconds (s), for example:

- A trampolinist performing a seat drop rotates their legs clockwise about the transverse axis 1.57 radians in 0.5 seconds. The average angular velocity is 3.14 rad/s (1.57 rad/0.5s).

Study hint

Angular speed and angular velocity are largely interchangeable. They are both measures of the rate of rotation; however, angular velocity also indicates a direction of spin, e.g. clockwise or anti-clockwise.

Study hint

If you are required to make a calculation in the exam, always show the formula you are using, your full workings and the units of measurement to gain some credit if the final calculation is incorrect.

Activity

The following data show the angular velocities over time of a gymnast performing a backward tucked somersault from take-off to landing.

Time taken (s)	0.00	0.05	0.10	0.15	0.20	0.25	0.30	0.35	0.40	0.45	0.50
Angular velocity (rad/s)	0.0	6.0	12.0	17.5	21.5	24.0	25.0	24.0	21.0	13.0	4.0

Using the data, draw a graph of angular velocity (vertical axis) against time taken (horizontal axis) for the somersault and explain the curve produced.

IN THE NEWS

After the widespread criticism Adidas received for the Jabulani football used in the 2010 South Africa World Cup being too hard to control and unpredictable in the air, improvements had to be made for Brazil in 2014. Adidas has its own laboratories for testing and one of its machines relies on angular velocity. The robotic leg can be set to rotate about its axis at a specific angular velocity to impart the exact same force, in the exact same place, on the Brazuca ball. The ball's motion in flight can then be monitored for consistency.

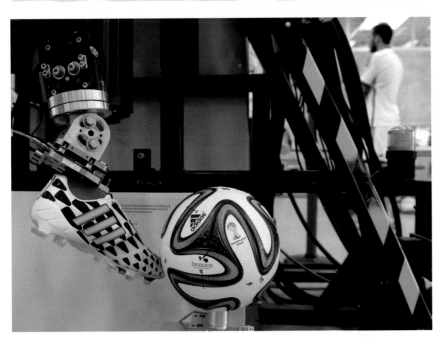

▲ Figure 3.2.6 The robotic leg imparting an eccentric force on the Brazuca ball at Adidas's testing laboratories

Moment of inertia

Moment of inertia (MI) is the resistance of a body to change its state of angular motion or rotation. A resting body will not want to start rotating around an axis and a rotating body will not want to change its angular motion or momentum; it will resist increasing or decreasing the rate of spin. Moment of inertia is the angular or rotational equivalent of inertia.

Key term

Moment of inertia: the resistance of a body to change its state of angular motion or rotation.

Moment of inertia can be calculated using the following equation:

Moment of inertia = sum of (mass × distribution of the mass from the axis of rotation^2)

$$MI = \Sigma\ m \times r^2$$

Moment of inertia is measured in kilogram metres^2 (kgm^2), mass in kilograms (kg) and distribution of the mass from the axis of rotation in metres^2 (m^2).

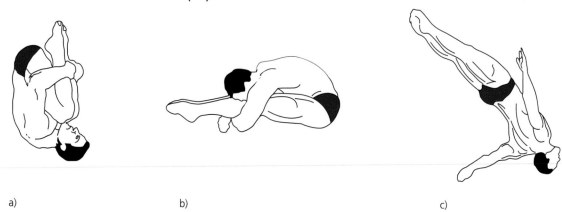

a)   b)   c)

▲ Figure 3.2.7 A high-board diver rotating around the transverse axis in varied positions: a) tucked somersault (MI low), b) piked somersault (MI moderate) and c) straight somersault (MI high)

The two factors that affect moment of inertia are mass and the distribution of mass from the axis of rotation.

- Mass. The greater the mass of a body, the greater the moment of inertia and vice versa. Sports with a high degree of rotation or technical requirement for complex twists and spins, such as high-board diving, gymnastics and dancing, are typically performed by athletes with a low mass.
  - The low mass decreases moment of inertia and the resistance to change state of rotation, so athletes can start rotation, change the rate of rotation and stop rotation with relative ease.
- Distribution of mass from the axis of rotation. The further the mass moves from the axis of rotation, the greater the moment of inertia and vice versa. Movements where the mass is tucked in around the axis of rotation, such as a front tucked somersault, a full twist or a scratch spin in ice skating, lower the moment of inertia.
  - The close 'tucked' mass distribution from the axis of rotation decreases moment of inertia and the resistance to change state of rotation. When performing a front tucked somersault the body will face less resistance to rotation and therefore rotate more quickly when compared with a straight somersault around the transverse axis.

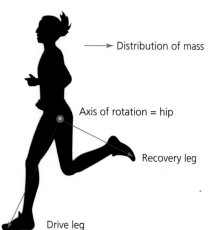

→ Distribution of mass

Axis of rotation = hip

Recovery leg

Drive leg

▲ Figure 3.2.8 The high moment of inertia of the drive leg compared with the low moment of inertia of the recovery leg during the running stride

When considering running technique, for example, both legs have the same mass and so should have the same moment of inertia. However:

- the recovery leg's mass is distributed close to the axis of rotation at the hip, therefore moment of inertia is low – resistance to rotation is low and the leg moves back to the ground quickly
- the drive leg's mass is distributed far from the axis of rotation at the hip, therefore moment of inertia is high – resistance to rotation is high and the leg moves slowly.

Based on this principle, sprint training will involve drills such as high knee lifts and heel flicks to encourage maximum bend (flexion) at the knee joint. This keeps the recovery leg close to the hip joint, rotating it quickly back to the ground.

Moment of inertia has a direct effect on angular velocity:

● If moment of inertia is high, resistance to rotation is also high, therefore angular velocity is low: the rate of spin is slow.

● If moment of inertia is low, resistance to rotation is also low, therefore angular velocity is high: the rate of spin is fast.

Moment of inertia throughout an action can be manipulated to perform complex movement patterns. For example, an ice skater performing a static spin on the ice will manipulate their body position to maximise the technicality of the spin and aesthetic appeal for the judges. Spinning around the longitudinal axis with body mass tucked into their body (bringing arms and legs closer to the midline of the body), the ice skater will reduce their moment of inertia, increasing angular velocity, and rotate very quickly. By moving their limbs away from the axis of rotation, the skater will increase their moment of inertia, reducing angular velocity, and decreasing the rate of spin.

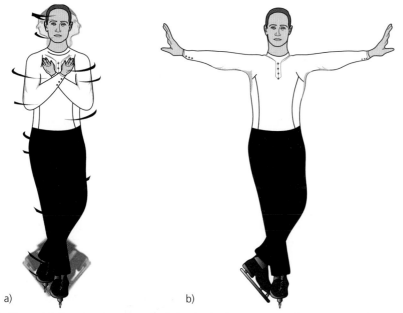

a)   b)

▲ Figure 3.2.9 An ice skater manipulating his body position to alter moment of inertia and angular velocity, a) low MI = fast rate of spin and b) high MI = slow rate of spin

Angular momentum

Angular momentum is the quantity of angular motion possessed by a body. It is the rotational equivalent of momentum and can be calculated using the following equation:

Angular momentum = moment of inertia × angular velocity

Angular momentum is measured in kilogram metres squared radians per second (kgm²rad/s), moment of inertia in kilogram metres squared (kgm²) and angular velocity in radians per second (rad/s), for example:

● A 60 kg gymnast performs a tucked front somersault. In the tucked phase their moment of inertia is 15 kgm² and they rotate with an

---

Activity

Can you think of any specific movements, techniques or actions that have a high and low moment of inertia in your sport? These can be of a specific limb, the whole body or a piece of equipment. Think about children learning technical movements. What is the easiest way to learn a forward roll, to start in a tucked-up ball or to take a running dive into the roll?

Activity

Apply the concept of moment of inertia to the different phases of the arm cycle in the freestyle (front crawl) stroke. Compare the moment of inertia in the propulsive phase as the arm enters the water to the high elbow in the recovery phase as the arm leaves the water.

Activity

You will need access to a freely rotating chair (computer chair) for this activity. In pairs, person one: sit down with limbs away from the longitudinal axis of rotation. Person two: spin the chair and let go. Person one: experiment what happens when the limbs move closer to and further from the longitudinal axis.

Key term

Angular momentum: the quantity of angular motion possessed by a body.

angular velocity of 8.0 rad/s. Their angular momentum in the tucked phase is 120 kgm²rad/s (15 kgm² × 8.0 rad/s).

To start rotating around an axis, angular momentum must be generated. In the preparation or take-off phase of a rotational movement pattern, an eccentric force or torque must be applied. For example, a high-board diver must jump away from the diving board and create rotation. They lean away from the board at take-off so the reaction force generated from the diving platform passes outside their centre of mass (they lean back to create a spinning effect). This creates an eccentric force and generates angular momentum. The greater the size of eccentric force applied to the body, the greater the quantity of angular momentum generated for the movement.

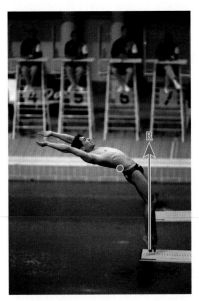

▲ Figure 3.2.10 Diver leaning away from the board at take-off to generate angular momentum

Extend your knowledge

Newton's laws of motion have angular 'versions' known as analogues. The angular analogue of Newton's second law of motion can be applied to the creation of angular momentum. It states: 'The rate of change in angular momentum of a body is directly proportional to the size of the eccentric force (or torque) applied and takes place in the same direction as the eccentric force is applied.'

Therefore, the greater the eccentric force applied to the diver at take-off from the board, the greater the rate of change in angular momentum generated and angular acceleration of the diver away from the board into the air. The effect is to gain a greater quantity of angular motion and perform more twists, spins and rotations in the time available.

Conservation of angular momentum

Once angular momentum has been generated it is a product of moment of inertia and angular velocity. As moment of inertia increases, angular velocity decreases and vice versa. This means angular momentum once generated does not change throughout a movement; it remains constant and therefore is termed a 'conserved' quantity. This means a performer can keep a rotation going for a long period of time, such as an ice skater performing a flat spin on the ice increasing and decreasing their rate of spin for dramatic effect, or a high-board diver rotating continuously until entry to the water.

The **conservation of angular momentum** is a concept associated with the **angular analogue of Newton's first law of motion**. This is the rotational equivalent of Newton's first law and states: 'A rotating body will continue to turn about its axis of rotation with constant angular momentum unless acted upon by an eccentric force or external torque.'

Study hint

When describing or applying the angular analogue of Newton's first law of motion, remember to state the key words 'axis of rotation', 'angular momentum' and 'torque' to show the difference between the angular analogue of Newton's first law of motion and Newton's first law of motion.

As angular momentum cannot be changed once in flight it is essential to generate as much angular momentum as possible at take-off. Once angular momentum has been generated the performer can then manipulate moment of inertia and therefore angular velocity to maximise their performance by including as many complex twists, spins and turns as possible to gain technical points.

So how would the conservation of angular momentum be applied to a sporting example? First, the axis of rotation should be considered, and second, the phases of motion the performer moves through, for example:

- the preparation, execution and recovery phases of a slalom skier rotating around the longitudinal axis as they rotate around the slalom pole
- the take-off, flight and landing phases of a trampolinist rotating around their transverse axis in a front somersault.

Finally, the key descriptors of angular motion – moment of inertia, angular velocity and angular momentum – should be described through each phase of motion. All three sections – axis of rotation, phases of motion and angular motion descriptors – come together to give a detailed explanation of how to perform a sporting movement with spin.

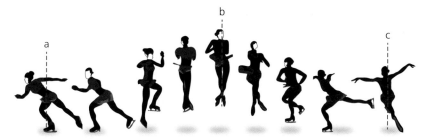

▲ Figure 3.2.11 Angular momentum remains constant about the longitudinal axis throughout flight when performing a triple axel jump in ice skating

Figure 3.2.11 shows an ice skater performing a triple axel jump with spin.

- Picture a shows how at take-off the ice skater generates angular momentum by applying an eccentric force from the ice to their body.
- The ice skater starts rotation about the longitudinal axis.
- Their distribution of mass is away from the longitudinal axis as their arms and one leg are held away from the midline. The moment of inertia is high and therefore angular velocity is low. They go into the jump rotating slowly and with control.
- Picture b shows how during flight the ice skater distributes their mass close to the longitudinal axis as they tuck in their arms and legs. The moment of inertia is decreased and therefore angular velocity is increased. They spin quickly, allowing several rotations in the time available in the air.
- Picture c shows how in preparation to land the ice skater distributes their mass away from the longitudinal axis, opening out the arms and one leg. The moment of inertia is raised and angular velocity reduced. They decrease their rate of spin, increasing their control for landing and preventing over-rotation.
- As they land, the ice applies an external torque to remove the conserved quantity of angular momentum maintained throughout the jump to move away smoothly.

Study hint

Don't forget to state the axis of rotation and don't worry if it feels as though you are repeating yourself – it is important to get across the theoretical concept at every stage.

Activity

Skate boarding, inline skating, snowboarding and skiing all use the same principles to perform stunts and tricks. Watch videos of skateboarder Tony Hawk's 900, snowboarder Shaun White's triple cork in a half pipe and aerial skier Jeret Peterson's back/full triple full-full jump. Discuss the concept of the conservation of angular momentum for each scenario. Some potential sporting applications are shown in the table below.

Axes of rotation	Sporting example to discuss the conservation of angular momentum
Longitudinal	A slalom skier rotating around the pole to change direction An ice skater performing a jump with spin
Transverse	A gymnast performing a front or back tucked somersault A diver performing a tucked front or backward somersault
Frontal	A side somersault on the beam in gymnastics

Extend your knowledge

If you like extreme sports, watch a video of Travis Pastrana at the X Games performing a double backflip in freestyle motorcross and explain why this would be so hard in terms of moment of inertia, angular velocity and angular momentum. (Consider the mass and potential to change the distribution of mass during the jump.)

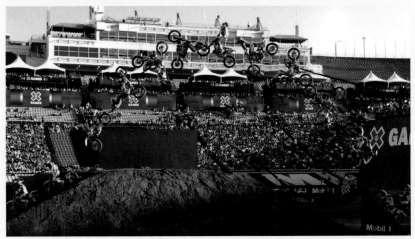

▲ Figure 3.2.12 Travis Pastrana's double backflip in freestyle motorcross

The key descriptors of angular motion can be recorded and plotted on a graph to represent the angular momentum of a movement pattern being performed. This graph can be used to gain a quick visual representation of complex data, identify the relationship between moment of inertia and angular velocity, and calculate angular momentum.

Study hint

For graphs of moment of inertia and/or angular velocity, always:
- plot time on the horizontal axis
- label the axes, including units in brackets
- use a curved line of best fit.

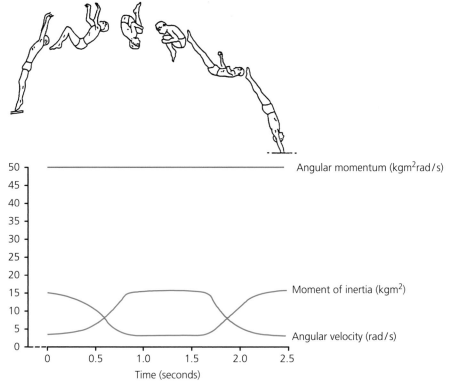

50 ——————————————————————— Angular momentum (kgm²rad/s)
45
40
35
30
25
20
15 ——————————————————— Moment of inertia (kgm²)
10
5 ——————————————————— Angular velocity (rad/s)
0
  0   0.5   1.0   1.5   2.0   2.5
        Time (seconds)

▲ Figure 3.2.13 The relationship between moment of inertia, angular velocity and angular momentum of a diver performing a one-and-a-half backward rotation into the water

Figure 3.2.13 shows a springboard diver performing a one-and-a-half backward rotation into the water. In comparison with the ice skater performing a jump with spin around the longitudinal axis, the diver rotates around the transverse axis:

- At take-off the diver generates angular momentum by an eccentric force from the springboard acting on the body (angular momentum = 50 kgm²rad/s) and starts rotation about the transverse axis.
- The straight body position distributes mass away from the transverse axis. The moment of inertia is high (15 kgm²) and angular velocity is low (3.3 rad/s). The diver rotates slowly and goes into the dive with control.
- During flight the diver's tucked body position distributes mass close to the transverse axis. Moment of inertia is decreased and angular velocity increased. The diver rotates quickly, enabling one-and-a-half rotations in the flight time.
- Preparing to land, the diver's straightened body position distributes mass away from the transverse axis. Moment of inertia is increased and angular velocity decreased. The rate of spin decreases, gaining control for entry to the water.
- Angular momentum is conserved throughout the movement.

Study hint

To impress in extended answers, try to use subject-specific vocabulary and fully explain your answers. For example, instead of 'the diver tucks in to spin quickly in the air' try 'in the flight phase the diver has a tucked position to distribute the mass close to the transverse axis of rotation. This will decrease the moment of inertia and increase the rate of spin, allowing more rotations.'

Study hint

Remember, a low moment of inertia is due to a low mass and/or a close distribution of mass to the axis of rotation: this causes a high angular velocity. When ice skaters, gymnasts or divers tuck in, it's to help them spin quickly.

Activity

Choose a sporting action such as a gymnastic tucked front somersault or slalom skier rotating about a pole and work through each phase of motion, describing moment of inertia, angular velocity and angular momentum.

Summary

Angular motion is movement in a circular path about an axis of rotation. It is a result of an eccentric force being applied to a body to create rotation around an axis, which can be measured, plotted and analysed to improve performance:

- There are three axes of rotation, imaginary lines that pass through the centre of mass about which a performer can rotate: the longitudinal axis, the transverse axis and the frontal axis.
- Angular velocity is the rate of change in angular displacement and can be calculated using: angular velocity = angular displacement/time taken (rad/s).
- Moment of inertia is the resistance of a body to change its state of angular motion or rotation and can be calculated: moment of inertia = sum of (mass × distribution of the mass from the axis of rotation^2). It is measured in kgm^2.
- Angular momentum is the quantity of angular motion possessed by a body and a product of moment of inertia and angular velocity. It is measured in kgm^{2}rad/s. When moment of inertia is high, angular velocity is low and vice versa; therefore, angular momentum remains constant.
- The angular analogue of Newton's first law of motion governs the conservation of angular momentum, stating: 'a rotating body will continue to turn about its axis of rotation with constant angular momentum unless acted upon by an eccentric force or external torque'.

Check your understanding

1 Answer the following statements as true or false:
   a An eccentric force is created when an external force passes outside a body's centre of mass.
   b A gymnast performing a cartwheel rotates around the frontal axis.
   c An ice skater rotates around the transverse axis when performing a jump with spin.
   d A radian is a unit of measurement showing the angular displacement of a body.
   e Moment of inertia is the resistance of a body to change its state of linear motion.
   f Moment of inertia is affected by a body's mass and the distribution of mass about the axis of rotation.
   g Angular momentum is the product of moment of inertia and angular velocity.
   h Angular momentum is a conserved quantity which increases and decreases throughout a movement.

2 Identify the key terms from the following statements:
   a Circular motion about an axis of rotation.
   b A measure of the turning or rotational force applied to a body.
   c The axis of rotation about which a slalom skier rotates when moving around a pole.
   d The rate of change in angular displacement (rad/s).
   e A rotating body will continue to turn about its axis of rotation with constant angular momentum unless acted upon by an eccentric force or external torque.

Practice questions

1 Define angular motion. Using a sporting example, explain how angular motion is created. Use a diagram to illustrate your answer. (3 marks)

2 Using sporting examples, explain the difference between planes of movement and axes of rotation. (4 marks)

3 State the angular analogue of Newton's first law of motion and apply it to a sporting situation. (4 marks)

4 Select either the transverse or the longitudinal axis of rotation and, using a sporting example of your choice, explain how a performer can manipulate their body position to control angular velocity. (6 marks)

3.3 Fluid mechanics and projectile motion

Understanding the specification

By the end of this chapter you should be able to demonstrate knowledge and understanding of fluid mechanics and projectile motion and how they can be manipulated in physical activity and sport:

- factors that affect air resistance and drag
- factors that affect horizontal distance travelled by a projectile
- free body diagrams and the resolution of forces acting on a projectile in flight
- parabolic and non-parabolic flight paths
- lift force, angle of attack and the Bernoulli principle
- spin and the Magnus effect.

Fluid mechanics

Fluid mechanics is the study of the forces acting on a body travelling through the air or water and so has particular importance for athletes in all sports.

- The force of **air resistance** acts on a body travelling at high velocity through the air, such as a cyclist, sprinter, skier, discus or shuttle.
- The force of **drag** acts on a body travelling through the water, such as a swimmer.

Air resistance and drag act in opposition to the direction of motion of the moving body and therefore must be minimised to perfect technique and performance. A huge amount of money is spent and research performed each year using wind tunnels and fluid dynamics programmes to analyse the effects of air resistance and drag in a bid to create the best equipment, clothing and coaching techniques. The UK has developed a leading reputation in Formula 1 and track cycling mechanics.

> **Key terms**
>
> **Air resistance:** the force that opposes the direction of motion of a body through the air.
> **Drag:** the force that opposes the direction of motion of a body through the water.

Magnitude of air resistance and drag

An athlete wants to put all of their energy into maximising performance and not waste it overcoming forces that hold them back. Air resistance and drag act against the motion of a body and place an increased physiological demand, which can lead to early fatigue and poor performance. By altering body position, equipment design and clothing an athlete can minimise air resistance and drag and gain a significant advantage.

There are four main factors that affect the magnitude of air resistance and drag on a body:

1   Velocity. The greater the velocity, the greater the air resistance or drag. Track cycling, speed skating, downhill skiing, a hard-hit shuttle and freestyle swimming are all greatly affected due to the high velocities travelled. Velocity cannot be reduced to minimise air resistance or drag and therefore other factors must be considered.

2   Frontal cross-sectional area. The larger the frontal cross-sectional area, the larger the air resistance or drag. Sports such as track cycling and downhill skiing are greatly affected due to the large frontal cross-section of the body facing the oncoming air. Every effort is made to reduce the size of the frontal cross-section to minimise air resistance and drag.

3   **Streamlining** and shape. The more streamlined or aerodynamic the shape of the body in motion, the lower the air resistance or drag. Streamlining is the creation of a smooth air flow around an aerodynamic shape. The more aerodynamic the shape of a body or equipment, the lower air resistance or drag will be. Many sports use a tear-drop or **aerofoil** shape, such as a track cyclist, downhill skier or speed skater's helmet.

4   Surface characteristics. The smoother the surface, the lower the air resistance or drag. Participants in sports such as swimming, cycling, sprinting, speed skating and skiing wear specially engineered clothing to create the smoothest surface possible to reduce the friction between the fluid and the body surface.

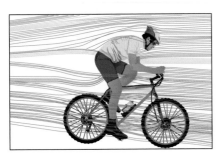

▲ Figure 3.3.1 Assessment of the air flow around a cyclist

Key terms

Streamlining: the creation of smooth air flow around an aerodynamic shape.

Aerofoil: a streamlined shape with a curved upper surface and flat lower surface designed to give an additional lift force to a body.

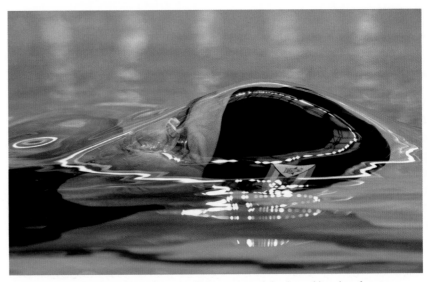

▲ Figure 3.3.2 Backstroke swimmer utilising a smooth body and head surface to minimise drag in the water

Consider the sport of downhill skiing. Elite male skiers can achieve velocities in excess of 40 metres per second (90 mph). With masses around 90 kg they generate a huge amount of momentum. As velocity is so high, downhill skiers must battle air resistance to maximise performance. They:

- minimise the frontal cross-sectional area by adopting a low crouched position in the straights and jump sections
- wear tear-drop-shaped helmets, and have fins on their gloves and around their boots to create a streamlined shape, easing the air flow around their body
- wear super silky Lycra suits to create a smooth surface.

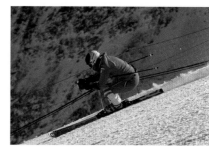

▲ Figure 3.3.3 Ski racer adopting a crouched position to reduce their frontal cross-sectional area

IN THE NEWS

US ski clothing maker Spyder created the 'tripwire' suit with wires running through the arms and legs, contouring air flow and reducing air resistance by 20 per cent. However, after complaints the suit wasn't available to all it was banned by the international federation. Spyder now uses wind tunnels in San Diego, with US ski team members subjected to wind speeds upwards of 80 mph to develop the best fabrics for air-resistance reduction. Fabric made as slippery as possible, suits with as few seams as possible and separate layers of thinner, smoother padding have led to 18 per cent less air resistance when compared with the previous Spyder giant slalom suit. This could translate into a several-second advantage in a giant slalom race.

Track cycling is another sport where huge advances have been made in terms of fluid mechanics. Cyclists travel at high velocities around the velodrome and suffer at the hands of air resistance. Team GB takes every step to optimise the bike, equipment, body position and team tactics to minimise air resistance, such as:

- lightweight carbon fibre bicycle design with aerodynamic features such as disc wheels and aerodynamic forks to reduce energy expenditure and minimise air resistance
- aerodynamic riding positions with shoulders forward, a high seat position to tilt the body forwards and narrow handlebars to bring in the hands and elbows to ensure a small frontal cross-sectional area
- aerodynamic helmets with a glossy surface and specialised shape to streamline air flow
- tight-fitting Lycra skin suits and smooth socks pulled over the shoes to seamlessly mould to the lower leg, and shaved legs, face and hands to maximise a smooth surface.

Activity

Consider the sport of swimming and drag in the water. Compare the different strokes and the manipulation of body position in the water, clothing and velocities achieved in relation to drag. Research the Speedo's LZR suit and newer clothing alternatives. Consider the role of technology in sport and official regulations to ensure all swimmers have a level playing field.

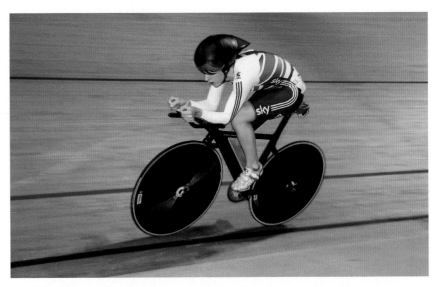

▲ Figure 3.3.4 Laura Trott of Team GB competing in the women's omnium individual pursuit at the track cycling World Championships in 2015

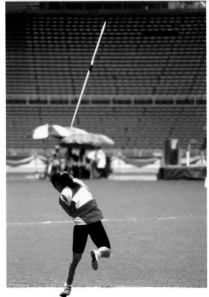

▲ Figure 3.3.5 The javelin becomes a projectile and starts its flight path after release

Extend your knowledge

Differences in air temperature and altitude also affect air resistance, which is of great importance in sports such as football as the distance of passes and spin placed on the ball will be affected. As air temperature increases, its density decreases, which reduces air resistance. As altitude increases, its density also decreases, which reduces air resistance. This can greatly impact on sports performance. For example, speed skaters can travel at speeds over 13 metres per second (30 mph) and be subjected to high levels of air resistance. All world records in races over 12 minutes' duration were set at tracks over 1,000 m altitude. In 2015 scientist Noordhof and colleagues found a 1,000 m increase in altitude resulted in performance improvements of 2.8 per cent in junior and 2.1 per cent in senior long-track speed skaters.

Projectile motion

Projectile motion is the movement of a body through the air following a curved flight path under the force of gravity. A **projectile** is a body launched into the air and subjected to weight and air resistance forces. Projectiles can be an athlete, such as a high jumper, or equipment that an athlete may throw, hit or kick, such as a javelin or tennis ball. Once in flight a projectile follows a flight path through the air. The flight path from start to finish shows the overall distance travelled after gravity has accelerated it back to the ground surface.

Projectile release

The flight path a projectile takes can be represented by a simple graph of height against horizontal distance travelled. This will give a quick visual impression of the shape of the flight path and overall distance travelled. It will also give an indication of the factors that have affected the flight path. The horizontal distance travelled by a projectile is primarily affected by four factors:

- speed of release
- angle of release
- height of release
- aerodynamic factors (Bernoulli and Magnus).

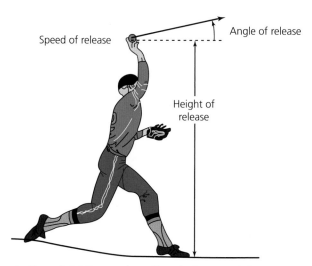

▲ Figure 3.3.6 Factors that affect the horizontal distance a projectile travels

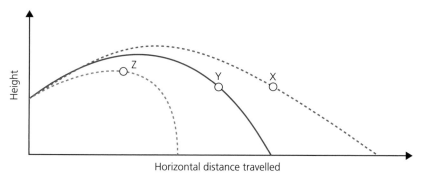

▲ Figure 3.3.7 The flight path of a hard-hit shuttle in badminton (Z), a shot in athletics (Y) and a tennis ball with backspin (X)

Speed of release

The horizontal distance a projectile travels is primarily affected by the speed of release. Due to Newton's second law of acceleration, the greater the force applied to the projectile, the greater the change in momentum and therefore acceleration of the projectile into the air. The greater the outgoing speed of the projectile, the further it will travel. Therefore, Olympic throwers will train to generate maximum power from their muscle mass in the arm, shoulder and chest region.

Angle of release

The horizontal distance a projectile travels is also affected by the angle of release. Based on a projectile being released at the same speed from the ground, at a release angle of:

- 90°: the projectile will accelerate vertically upwards and come straight back down, travelling 0 m
- 45°: optimal angle to maximise horizontal distance
- greater than 45°, such as 60° or 75°: the projectile reaches peak height too quickly and rapidly returns to the ground
- less than 45°, such as 30°: the projectile does not achieve sufficient height to maximise flight time.

Activity

Experiment with the speed, angle and height of release and horizontal distance a projectile can travel. For ease simply use a ball of paper and bin placed above, below and at the same height you throw or kick from. Work in groups and discuss your findings.

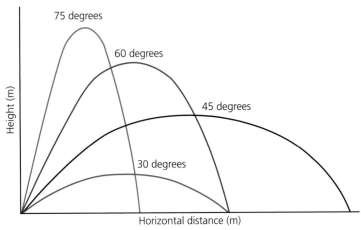

▲ Figure 3.3.8 Angle of release and horizontal distance travelled

Height of release

45° is the optimal angle of release if the release height and landing height are equal. However, if the height of projectile release is higher or lower than the landing height, the optimal angle will change. For example:

- where the release height is above the landing height (positive relative release height) – for example, in the javelin and shot – the optimal angle of release is less than 45° as the projectile already has an increased flight time due to the increased height of release
- where the release height is below the landing height (negative relative release height) – for example, a bunker shot in golf – the optimal angle of release is more than 45° as the projectile needs an increased flight time to overcome the obstacle.

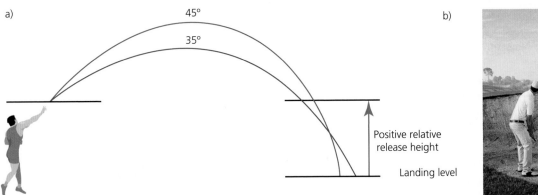

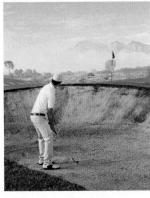

▲ Figure 3.3.9 Height of release will affect the optimal angle of release for maximum horizontal distance of a projectile, a) a shot putter's height of release is above the landing height, b) a golf bunker shot's height of release is below the landing height

Projectiles in flight

Flight path

Once released, a projectile follows a flight path determined by the relative size of the forces acting upon it. The true flight path of a projectile unaffected by air resistance mirrors the mathematical shape of a **parabola**, a uniform curve symmetrical about its highest point. Flight paths are described relative to a parabolic shape. In flight a projectile is affected by weight and air resistance. Depending on the dominant force, the flight path will be more or less parabolic in nature:

- If weight is the dominant force and air resistance is very small, a **parabolic flight path** occurs.
  - For example, a shot put has a very high mass and travels through the air at a low velocity, with a relatively small frontal cross-sectional area and smooth surface, which makes air resistance negligible.
  - The flight path has a parabolic shape symmetrical about its highest point.
- If air resistance is the dominant force and weight is very small, a **non-parabolic flight path** occurs.
  - For example, a badminton shuttle has a very low mass and travels at high velocities with a relatively uneven surface, which all increase air resistance.
  - The flight path has a non-parabolic shape asymmetrical (unequal) about its highest point.

As the effect of air resistance increases, the more a projectile will deviate from a parabolic flight path.

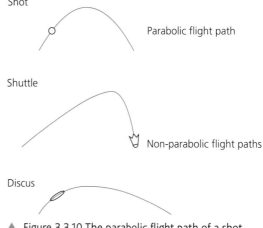

▲ Figure 3.3.10 The parabolic flight path of a shot compared with the non-parabolic flight paths of a shuttle and discus

> **Key terms**
>
> **Parabola:** a uniform curve symmetrical about its highest point.
> **Parabolic flight path:** a flight path symmetrical about its highest point caused by the dominant weight force of a projectile.
> **Non-parabolic flight path:** a flight path asymmetrical about its highest point caused by the dominant force of air resistance on the projectile.

Free body diagrams

The forces acting on a projectile in flight can be represented with a **free body diagram**. This is a simple sketch to give a snapshot of the forces acting on a body at a specific moment in time. The free body diagram will show which forces are acting, where the forces originate, the relative sizes of the forces and the direction in which they are acting on the projectile. This will allow us to consider the net force acting on the body and therefore the resulting projectile motion and flight path.

There are three phases of motion within a flight path to the highest point after which gravity will accelerate the projectile's mass to the ground. These can be described as:

- start of flight
- mid flight
- end of flight.

Over these phases weight force does not change, whereas air resistance may be dependent on the velocity of the moving projectile, such as a hard-hit shuttle in badminton. Air resistance will be far greater at the start of flight after release as it is travelling with the highest velocity. This will cause rapid deceleration of the shuttle in flight, consequently reducing air resistance until its highest point. At the highest point weight becomes a more dominant force. Overall, the flight path is non-parabolic.

> **Key term**
>
> **Free body diagram:** a clearly labelled sketch showing all of the forces acting on a body at a particular instant in time.

> **Activity**
>
> Draw a flight path diagram to represent the flight path of an athletics shot in flight. Annotate the diagram, explaining what shape the flight path is and why. Draw three free body diagrams showing the forces acting on the shot at the start, middle and end of flight. This is different from Figure 3.3.11 of the badminton shuttle on the next page: why?

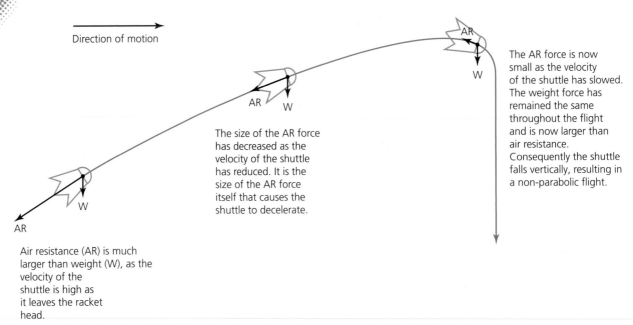

Direction of motion

The AR force is now small as the velocity of the shuttle has slowed. The weight force has remained the same throughout the flight and is now larger than air resistance. Consequently the shuttle falls vertically, resulting in a non-parabolic flight.

The size of the AR force has decreased as the velocity of the shuttle has reduced. It is the size of the AR force itself that causes the shuttle to decelerate.

Air resistance (AR) is much larger than weight (W), as the velocity of the shuttle is high as it leaves the racket head.

▲ Figure 3.3.11 Free body diagrams of a shuttle in the start-, mid- and end-of-flight phases

Study hint

When drawing a free body diagram, keep it simple. Use a simple shape to represent the projectile and identify the weight and air resistance forces acting at the moment described in the question. In addition:
- weight and air resistance should originate from the centre of mass of the projectile
- weight should project downwards
- air resistance should project opposite to the direction of motion
- always include a direction-of-motion arrow.

Table 3.3.1 Free body diagrams mid-flight and flight paths of a) a shot in athletics compared with b) a hard-hit badminton shuttle

	Free body diagram	Dominant force	Resulting flight path
Shot	(a) Air resistance ← ● → Direction of motion ↓ Weight	Weight > Air resistance	Parabolic
Shuttle	(b) Air resistance ← ⬦ → Direction of motion ↓ Weight	Air resistance > Weight	Non-parabolic

Parallelogram of forces

To consider the result of all forces acting on a projectile in flight, a **parallelogram of forces** can be drawn. This diagram uses the parallelogram law to show the **resultant force** acting on the projectile (sum of all forces acting or net force) and is created by:

- drawing a free body diagram showing the forces of weight and air resistance
- adding broken parallel lines to the weight and air resistance arrows to create the parallelogram

- drawing a diagonal line from the origin of weight and air resistance (the centre of mass of the projectile) to the opposite corner of the parallelogram with a double arrow labelled 'resultant force'.

The resultant force shows the acceleration of a projectile and the direction in which the acceleration occurs. The resultant force will also indicate the flight path:

- If the resultant force is closer to the weight arrow, the force of weight is dominant and therefore the flight path will be more parabolic in nature. This will be shown in a parallelogram of forces diagram of a shot put in flight.

- If the resultant force is closer to the air resistance arrow, the force of air resistance is dominant and therefore the flight path will be non-parabolic in nature. This will be shown in a parallelogram of forces diagram of a hard-hit shuttle in flight.

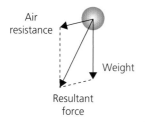

The resultant force shows deceleration to be occurring and weight to be dominant, leading to a parabolic flight path

▲ Figure 3.3.12 Parallelogram of forces for a shot mid-flight showing the resultant force

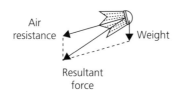

The resultant force shows deceleration to be occurring and air resistance to be dominant, leading to a non-parabolic flight path

▲ Figure 3.3.13 Parallelogram of forces for a badminton shuttle mid-flight showing the resultant force

Evaluation

- If weight is dominant, the flight path is more parabolic.
- If air resistance is dominant, the flight path is more non-parabolic.
- A free body diagram shows all forces acting on a projectile in flight.
- The parallelogram law shows the resultant force acting on the projectile in flight.

Study hint

Do not create a parallelogram on the same free body diagram you have drawn to show all the forces acting on a projectile in flight. Draw a second diagram to ensure you access all marks available.

Lift and the Bernoulli principle

Being able to manipulate the flow of air around a projectile can be of great advantage in the sporting field. Daniel Bernoulli, a professor of mathematics in the eighteenth century, applied his understanding of fluid dynamics to create the principle of 'lift' that is now critical to product design and sporting technique.

The **Bernoulli principle** is the underlying theory of how an additional **lift force** can be created during flight based on the shape of a projectile. The overall effect of additional lift is to increase the time the projectile hangs in the air, extending the flight path and horizontal distance covered. This can lead to better results in events such as throwing the discus and javelin and ski jumping.

Activity

Hold a single piece of A4 paper (portrait) in two corners up to your mouth. In a long, slow breath, blow along the upper surface of the paper and observe what happens. Relate it to the underlying theory of the Bernoulli principle.

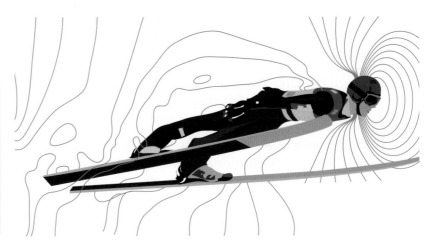

▲ Figure 3.3.14 A ski jumper in flight adopting an aerofoil shape

An aerofoil shape has a curved upper surface and flat underneath surface, as seen in the cross section of an aeroplane wing. As the aerofoil moves through the air it is forced to part and flow at different velocities above and below the projectile to meet at the same time behind. This affects the pressure of air flow above and below the aerofoil and a pressure gradient forms, generating an additional force:

- The curved upper surface forces air flow to travel a further distance and therefore move at a higher velocity.
- The flat underneath surface allows air to flow a shorter distance and therefore at a comparatively lower velocity.

As velocity increases, pressure decreases:

- Above the curved upper surface, a low-pressure zone is created.
- Below the flat underneath surface, a high-pressure zone is created.

Key term

Angle of attack: the most favourable angle of release for a projectile to optimise lift force due to the Bernoulli principle.

As all fluids move from an area of high to low pressure, a pressure gradient forms, creating an additional lift force. This is utilised by a ski jumper who leaves the ramp and adopts the aerofoil shape in the air with flat skis forming the underneath surface and the head and back forming the curved upper surface (as shown in Figure 3.3.14).

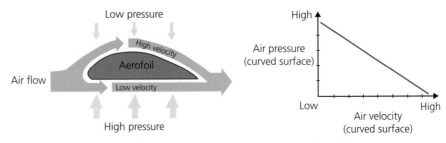

▲ Figure 3.3.15 Air flow, velocity and pressure around an aerofoil in flight

To fully explain the effect of the Bernoulli principle on a projectile in sport, several diagrams can be used. Using the example of throwing the discus in athletics, the discus becomes a projectile launched at an optimal **angle of attack** of 17° to act as an aerofoil to maximise Bernoulli's lift force in flight. An air flow diagram will illustrate this concept – see Figure 3.3.16.

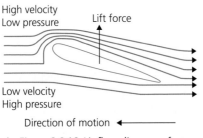

▲ Figure 3.3.16 Air flow diagram of a discus in flight

To demonstrate the effects of Bernoulli's lift force on the flight of the discus, three further diagrams can be drawn (see Figure 3.3.17):

- A free body diagram to show all three forces acting on the discus: lift force, weight and air resistance.

- A resultant force diagram to show the sum of all forces acting on the discus using a parallelogram of forces. When drawing a resultant force diagram, the vertical forces must be resolved. The additional lift generated reduces the force of weight and is indicated by the label 'W – lift force'.

- A flight path diagram to show the effect on the horizontal distance the discus travels.

a)
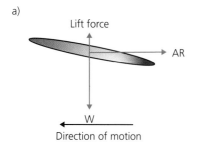

b)
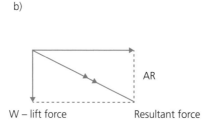

Note: Vertical forces are resolved: weight minus lift force. Resultant force shows the discus is decelerating in flight and closer to AR, therefore the flight path will be non-parabolic

c)
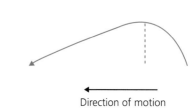

Note: Non-parabolic flight path. Extended horizontal distance travelled

▲ Figure 3.3.17 The effects of Bernoulli's lift force on a discus in flight: a) free body diagram, b) resultant force diagram and c) flight path diagram

Downward lift force

Bernoulli's lift force also works in a downward direction if the aerofoil shape is inverted. This has been used in sports such as Formula 1 and track cycling to increase the downward force that holds the car or bike to the track at high speeds around corners.

In Formula 1 the front wing funnels air down through the narrow space underneath the car's chassis and the spoiler bar acts as an inverted aerofoil, forcing air underneath it to travel a further distance. Both of these manipulations increase the velocity of air flow underneath the car and below the spoiler bar, creating areas of low pressure. A pressure gradient forms and an additional downward lift force is created, pinning the car to the track. This increases friction and grip around the corners at high speeds. In fact, this effect is so great that when a Formula 1 race car travels at speeds of around 120 mph the race track could be turned upside down and the car would stay attached to the surface.

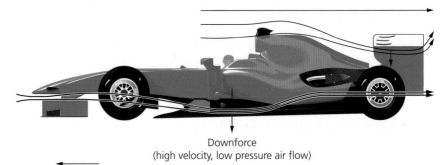

Downforce
(high velocity, low pressure air flow)

Direction of motion

▲ Figure 3.3.18 The downward lift force created by Formula 1 car design: air flow diagram with high velocity air flow and low pressure underneath the car and spoiler

Extend your knowledge

The Venturi effect followed on from the Bernoulli principle to show the increase in air flow velocity when a body of air is squeezed through a narrow space. Again this increase in velocity of air through a narrow space coincides with an area of low pressure, creating a pressure gradient and lift force. Formula 1 car designers utilise this by creating a Venturi underneath the car chassis to maximise downforce.

Activity

Apply Bernoulli's downward lift force to a track cyclist. Consider the high seat position and helmet design to create a flat back position, the forward rotation of the wheels and high knee lift. Draw an air flow diagram to illustrate where the oncoming body of air would move above and below the cyclist and the effects of the shape the air flow creates.

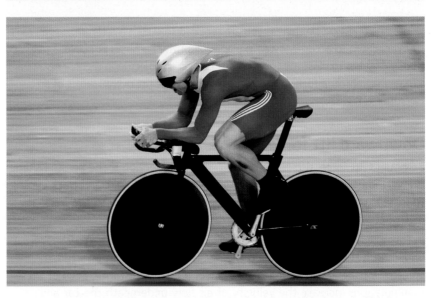

▲ Figure 3.3.19 Track cyclist Sir Chris Hoy benefits from Bernoulli's downward lift force

Spin and the Magnus force

Heinrich Magnus followed Bernoulli in the early nineteenth century to apply fluid mechanics to rotating projectiles. The **Magnus effect** is the underlying theory of how an additional **Magnus force** can deviate a spinning projectile away from its expected flight path. When used correctly this additional Magnus force can swerve a football around a wall, extend the flight of a golf drive or accelerate a topspin serve in tennis to mislead the opposition.

Spin is created by applying an external force outside the centre of mass. Where this eccentric force is applied will determine the way the projectile (usually a ball) spins. There are four types of spin:

- topspin: eccentric force applied above centre of mass (spins downwards around the transverse axis)
- backspin: eccentric force applied below centre of mass (spins upwards around the transverse axis)
- sidespin **hook**: eccentric force applied right of the centre of mass (spins left around the longitudinal axis)
- sidespin **slice**: eccentric force applied left of the centre of mass (spins right around the longitudinal axis).

Key terms

Magnus effect: creation of an additional Magnus force on a spinning projectile which deviates from the flight path.
Magnus force: a force created from a pressure gradient on opposing surfaces of a spinning body moving through the air.
Hook: a type of sidespin used to deviate a projectile's flight path to the left.
Slice: a type of sidespin used to deviate a projectile's flight path to the right.

Study hint

All explanations of sidespin are for a right-handed or right-footed player.

The Magnus effect works on the same theoretical basis as the Bernoulli principle. However, instead of a projectile's specific shape we consider the effect of the projectile's rotation or spin. The way the projectile spins determines the direction, velocity and pressure of air flow around it. Again a pressure gradient is formed either side of the spinning projectile and an additional Magnus force is created which deviates the flight path. This deviation means all forms of spin create a non-parabolic flight path:

- A topspin rotation creates a downward Magnus force, shortening the flight path.
- A backspin rotation creates an upward Magnus force, lengthening the flight path.
- A sidespin rotation creates a Magnus force to the right (slice) and left (hook), swerving the projectile right (slice) and left (hook).

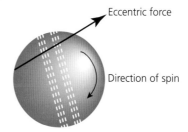

▲ Figure 3.3.20 Application of an eccentric force to impart topspin on a ball

For a ball with topspin the additional Magnus force is created by:

- the upper surface of the projectile rotating towards the oncoming air flow (top to bottom), which opposes motion, decreasing the velocity of air flow – a high pressure zone is created
- the lower surface of the projectile rotating in the same direction as the air flow, which increases the velocity of air flow and creates a zone of low pressure
- a pressure gradient forming and an additional Magnus force being created downwards (all gases move from an area of high pressure to an area of low pressure).

The downward Magnus force adds to the weight of the projectile and the effect of gravity is increased. The projectile 'dips' in flight, giving less time in the air as the flight path shortens.

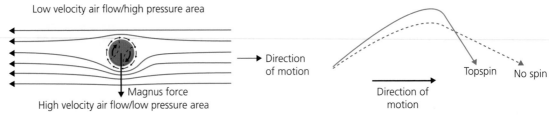

Low velocity air flow/high pressure area

Direction of motion

Magnus force
High velocity air flow/low pressure area

Topspin   No spin

Direction of motion

▲ Figure 3.3.21 Air flow diagram illustrating the downward Magnus force created by topspin

▲ Figure 3.3.22 Flight path diagram showing the effect of topspin

In tennis and table tennis, placing spin on the ball gives it stability in flight, guiding the air flow and reducing turbulence. The use of topspin shortens the flight path, meaning a player can hit the ball harder, thus ensuring it will still land in court or on the table; for example, a topspin serve in tennis or a topspin drive in table tennis. It can also confuse the opposition, bringing them closer to the net and unexpectedly putting them in a defensive position.

Activity

If an eccentric force is applied beneath the centre of mass, backspin is created. Explain how the additional Magnus force is created on a backspinning ball and how this is used to a player's advantage in tennis and table tennis. Use the following prompts to guide you and sketch diagrams to add to your explanation:
- upper surface of the ball (rotates in the same direction as air flow): effect on velocity and pressure
- underneath surface of the ball (opposes air flow): effect on velocity and pressure
- pressure gradient forms as all gases move from an area of high pressure to low pressure, creating the additional Magnus force: direction of Magnus force and effect on time in the air and length of flight path
- use of backspin in table tennis and tennis
- air flow and flight path diagram.

Free body and resultant force diagrams can also be drawn to show the forces acting on a spinning ball in flight and the resultant force using the parallelogram law. Biomechanists then use these diagrams to analyse performance of both athletes and equipment. Tiny changes in the surface of a ball, for example, can have a big impact in their flight through the air – for example, for a ball with backspin in flight.

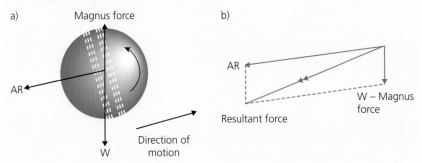

▲ Figure 3.3.23 a) Free body diagram showing the forces acting on a ball with backspin in flight and b) resultant force diagram showing the sum of all forces acting on a ball with backspin in flight

Study hint

When drawing an air flow diagram for a ball with topspin or backspin it is viewed from the side whereas sidespin is drawn from above. Air flow diagrams must show:
- direction of air flow opposing the direction of motion
- direction of rotation of the ball
- velocity and pressure labels
- more and tighter air flow lines with the direction of rotation side of the ball
- Magnus force in the direction of flight path deviation from the centre of mass.

Extend your knowledge

The effects of topspin and backspin in tennis extend to the bounce of the ball:
- A ball with topspin accelerates at a low angle on bounce as the friction with the ground surface acts in the same direction of motion. This advantages athletes with powerful serves, compact, short strokes and a variety of shots, such as Novak Djokovic, especially on the fastest surface: the grass courts of Wimbledon.
- A ball with backspin decelerates and bounces at a steep angle as the friction with the ground surface acts against the direction of the ball. This advantages agile athletes who can move across the whole court rapidly to return balls that 'sit up' after bounce, such as Rafael Nadal, especially on the loose surface clay courts of Roland Garros.

Sidespin is also well used for making a ball swerve in flight, both hook to the left and slice to the right. These types of spin can be viewed easily from above, as illustrated in air flow diagrams. Table 3.3.2 provides an overview of both hook and slice.

Table 3.3.2 An overview of a golf ball struck with sidespin, hook and slice

Type of sidespin	Air flow diagram	Description	Flight path diagram
Hook	Direction of travel. Magnus force. High velocity air flow/low pressure area. Low velocity air flow/high pressure area	• Air flow opposes motion. • Ball rotates to the left, guiding air flow (high velocity/low pressure). • Ball rotates against air flow on the right side, resisting air flow (low velocity/high pressure). • Pressure gradient formed. • Magnus force acts to deviate the flight path to the left.	No spin. Sidespin hook. Direction of motion
Slice	Direction of travel. Magnus force. Low velocity air flow/high pressure area. High velocity air flow/low pressure area	• Air flow opposes motion. • Ball rotates to the right, guiding air flow (high velocity/low pressure). • Ball rotates against air flow on the left side, resisting air flow (low velocity/high pressure). • Pressure gradient formed. • Magnus force acts to deviate the flight path to the right.	No spin. Sidespin slice. Direction of motion

In golf, placing sidespin on the ball will allow it to swerve in flight, moving the golf ball around obstacles in its path, such as trees or bends in the fairway. In tennis and table tennis, placing sidespin on the ball can confuse the opposition, moving them to the outside of the court or table unexpectedly after, for example, a topspin slice serve, giving the player an open court/table to go on the attack. However, it is most well appreciated on the football pitch. Sidespin is used to swerve a football around a wall when taking a free kick or into the goal mouth from a corner kick. This can produce quite spectacular results and create sporting icons such as David Beckham and Roberto Carlos, famous for their free kicks and goals from unenviable positions.

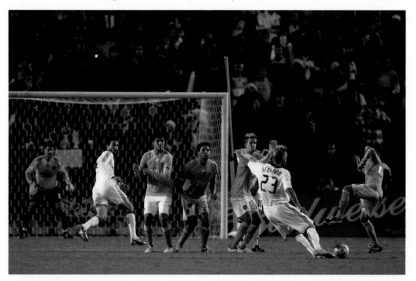

▲ Figure 3.3.24 Sidespin and the Magnus effect in action as David Beckham moves the ball around the wall and into the goal

Remember that the use of sporting examples is essential in this part of the course. Make sure you can link topspin and backspin to tennis and table tennis, and sidespin to tennis, table tennis, football and golf.

Extend your knowledge

A golf club and ball are in contact for approximately half a millisecond. During this time even the tiniest of differences in the direction the club faces can have a huge impact on the flight path of the golf ball. An elite golfer can swerve the ball around obstacles; however, a misalignment of just 1° is enough to cause the ball to swerve up to eight yards from a non-spinning path in the air by the end of a 200-yard drive, either hook to the left or slice to the right. A tilt in the club face of up to 3° can send the ball flying off into the rough at the side of the fairway.

Activity

Research the Adidas Jabulani football from the South Africa World Cup in 2010 and compare it with the performance of the redesigned Brazuca ball used in South America in 2014. Consider their performance, stability and reliability as a spinning projectile and their effect on the game for both players and spectators.

Summary

Fluid mechanics is the study of the forces acting on a body travelling through air or water. As a body moves through the air it may be subject to additional forces, all of which can be analysed and manipulated to improve performance:

- At high velocity, air resistance and fluid friction are significant and must be minimised by reducing frontal cross-sectional area, streamlining and smoothing the surface of an aerodynamic shape.
- Projectile motion is the movement of a body through the air. The horizontal distance a projectile travels is affected largely by speed, angle and height of release.
- In flight, if weight is dominant, a projectile's flight path will be more parabolic – for example, a shot put – whereas if air resistance is dominant, the flight path will be more non-parabolic – for example, a badminton shuttle.
- Using the Bernoulli principle, an additional lift force can be created by using an aerofoil shape in flight. This will increase the time the projectile hangs in the air, extending the flight path and horizontal distance covered:
  - A reverse aerofoil shows Bernoulli's lift force working in a downward direction to increase the friction with the track in Fomula1 and track cycling.
- Using the Magnus effect, an additional Magnus force can be created on a spinning projectile:
  - Topspin will dip the projectile and shorten the flight path.
  - Backspin will float the projectile and extend the flight path.
  - Sidespin will swerve the projectile to the left with a hook spin and to the right with a slice spin.

1 Answer the following statements as true or false:
 a Projectile motion is movement of a body through the air following a curved flight path under the force of gravity.
 b Streamlining is the creation of turbulent air flow behind an aerodynamic shape.
 c A non-parabolic flight path is symmetrical about its highest point.
 d An aerofoil is a streamlined shape created by a spinning projectile.
 e Horizontal distance travelled by a projectile is mainly affected by speed, angle and height of release.
 f The parallelogram law can be used to illustrate the resultant force acting on a projectile in flight.
 g The optimal angle of attack to launch a projectile to gain additional lift force is 17°.
 h There are two types of spin: topspin and backspin.

2 Identify the key terms from the following statements:
 a A force that opposes the direction of motion of a body through the air.
 b A body launched into the air losing contact with the ground.
 c A flight path symmetrical about its highest point caused by a dominance of weight.
 d The creation of lift force on a projectile in flight resulting from the relationship between air flow velocity and air pressure.
 e A force created from a pressure gradient on opposing surfaces of a spinning body moving through a fluid.

Practice questions

1 Explain how a 50 m freestyle swimmer reduces the fluid friction that acts against them in the water. (4 marks)

2 Define angle of attack and eccentric force and explain why these two terms are important for different types of projectile motion. (4 marks)

3 Using a sporting example, explain the use of topspin to alter the flight path of a ball in flight. (6 marks)

4 Discuss how a ski jumper minimises air resistance on their descent down the ramp and maximises the horizontal distance they travel in the jump. Use diagrams to help explain your answer where necessary. (20 marks)

Part 4
Skill acquisition

4.1 Memory models

4.1 Memory models

Atkinson and Shiffren's multi-store memory model

Memory is so important for sports performers, whether they are learning new skills or developing previously acquired skills and strategies. Remembering the correct techniques as well as the tactics required to be effective in sport is crucial to all sports performers. Most psychologists do not view memory as an entity, but rather a process involving the processing of information by the brain. The brain is viewed as actively altering and organising information rather than merely recording it. There are three stages of remembering information. This process was developed by Atkinson and Shiffren and is known as the multi-store memory model.

Encoding

This involves the conversion of information into codes called visual codes, auditory codes and semantic codes. The latter is the conversion of information according to meaning – for example, if we hear the coach tell us a tactical play in basketball, we may not remember it word for word, but we will remember the essential meaning.

Storage

This concerns the retention of information over a period of time.

Retrieval

This involves recovering the information that has been stored. The success of this retrieval depends on how well known the information is and how much there is of it.

The memory is very important in processing information. Our previous experiences affect how we judge and interpret information and the course of action we take.

The memory process is complex, and although there has been much research in this area, it is still not understood fully. However, simplified models such as the multi-store memory model have been developed to try to explain the process. The basic model describes memory as essentially a three-stage process: short-term sensory store → short-term memory → long-term memory (see Figure 4.1.1). All relevant information that is selected passes through the short-term memory. The process of **chunking** (organisation of information) can help a performer deal with larger amounts of information. Items of information need to be rehearsed before they can be stored in the long-term memory.

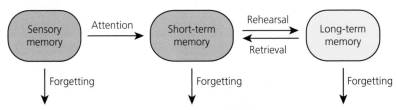

▲ Figure 4.1.1 Adapted from Atkinson and Shiffren's multi-store memory model

Key term

Chunking: different pieces of information can be grouped (or chunked) together and then remembered as one piece of information.

Short-term sensory stores

Information in the form of stimuli enters the brain from the environment. Each store has a large capacity, but information is stored for only between a quarter and one second before it is filtered. This filtering takes place in the stimulus identification stage. **Selective attention** takes place in the short-term sensory stores. This process is particularly important in sport, where quick reactions depend on being able to concentrate on important information and to shut out distractions.

Key term

Selective attention: relevant information is filtered through into the short-term memory and irrelevant information is lost or forgotten.

Short-term memory

This has been named the 'workspace' or the 'working memory' because this is where the information is used to decide what needs to be done. Only a limited amount of information can be stored in the short-term memory (research is ambiguous but points to about seven pieces of information) and it is held for only a brief time (about 30 seconds). To extend this time, the performer would have to rehearse the information, through imagery or sub-verbal repetition (by talking to yourself). Information can also be held in the short-term memory through a process called chunking. For example, instead of trying to remember each separate move made by each player in a line-out in rugby, or a penalty corner in hockey, a player might remember the whole drill as a single number.

If information is considered important enough and is rehearsed, it can be passed into the long-term memory. This process is called encoding the information. Information that is not considered important, or is not rehearsed, is usually lost because it does not go into the long-term memory.

Long-term memory

This store of information has almost limitless capacity and holds information for long periods of time. The stored information has been encoded. Information is stored in the long-term memory possibly by associating it with other information or with meaning. Meaningless items are usually not stored for long periods of time – for example, in swimming you may be aware of the depth notices on the side of the pool, but these may be largely meaningless to your performance in a swimming race. Motor programmes are stored in the long-term memory because they have been rehearsed many times. The process of continued rehearsal leads to a skill being almost automatic, and the process of learning by rehearsal is often referred to as 'overlearning'. If you are using particular motor skills

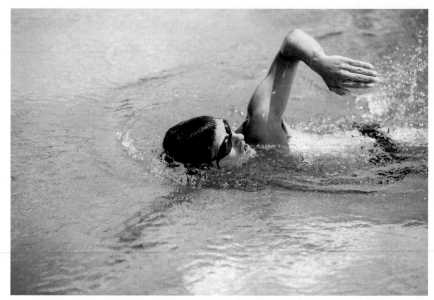

regularly, you are more likely to remember them – for example, once you have learned to swim, you are unlikely to forget. Recall of information passes from long-term memory back to short-term memory.

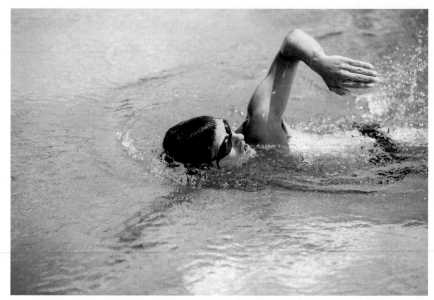

▲ Figure 4.1.2 Once you have learned to swim, you are unlikely to forget

Craik and Lockhart's levels of processing model

This approach, developed by Craik and Lockhart in 1972, is used to explain how memory works and opposes the view that there are set memory stores shown by the multi-store memory model. The levels of processing model seeks to explain what we do with the information rather than how it is stored. How deeply we consider or process information dictates how long the memory lasts.

Information received by the brain will be transferred to the long-term memory and therefore remembered more if the information:

- is considered
- is understood
- has meaning (related to past memories).

Therefore, according to this approach, the meaning of the information is much more relevant than mere repetition.

How much this information is considered is called the 'depth of processing'. The deeper the information is processed, the longer the memory or **memory trace** will last.

This approach identifies three possible levels related to the processing of verbal information:

1   Structural level – this involves paying attention to what the words look like. This is a shallow level of processing.

2   Phonetic level – this involves processing the sounds of words.

3   Semantic level – this considers the actual meaning of words, which is the deepest level of processing.

With the levels of processing approach to learning movement skills, instructions and demonstrations need to be able to show or elicit meaning from the activity – the more information means something to the performer, the more likely it is that they will remember it.

A practical example of this approach in action might be a gymnastics coach explaining why it is important to take a tuck position in a somersault to ensure greater speed in rotation. The performer is more likely to understand why she has to assume a tuck position and therefore more likely to remember this action.

Evaluation

The two memory approaches
The two approaches to explaining the memory process have both advantages and disadvantages that we can explore to be able to critically evaluate each approach.

Multi-store memory model
Advantages:
- Simplifies the memory process to aid understanding.
- Explains how those with brain damage may have dysfunctional memory or amnesia, showing a distinction between short-term and long-term memory.

Disadvantages:
- Too simplified – does not explain why we remember different types of information. For example, we might more easily remember a coach's explanation of a sports technique rather than a simplified diagram.
- Does not effectively prove the distinction between short-term memory and long-term memory and does not effectively explain the interaction between short-term and long-term memory.

Levels of processing approach
Advantages:
- Explains well that if we understand some information, we are more likely to remember it – coaches have often stated that they understand their sport more now because they have to explain its skills and strategies and therefore remember more clearly the coaching points to be made to performers.
- Explains well that the longer we consider and analyse information, the more we remember that information.

Disadvantages:
- The longer time it takes to process information does not always lead to better recall. So the depth of processing does not always help us to remember.
- Difficulty in defining what 'deep' processing actually involves. In merely describing the brain as processing information 'deeply', there is little to define what is meant by 'deeply'.
- Does not take into account individual differences. For instance, why do those who show more determination sometimes forget basic skills? Or why is it that those who pay little attention to the coach's instructions can perform so well and remember the coaching points and strategies that may lead to winning performances?

RESEARCH IN FOCUS

Research by Craik and Baddeley in the 1980s revealed that other aspects of how information is given or presented can affect how deep a performer's processing might be:

The 'elaboration' of information – if further explanation is given about why a movement is important, it is more likely that the performer will remember the action.

'Personal relevance' has been shown to be significant to memory – if the information and explanation from coaches relate movements to the performer's experiences, then the performer is more likely to retain the information. For example, when a gymnastics coach, addressing a dismount from the beam, refers the gymnast to a somersault they previously performed successfully, this may have more personal relevance to the gymnast, who is more likely to remember specific coaching points to improve performance.

The 'distinctiveness' of the information has also been identified as important to ensure that the processing of information is 'deep' – if the coach makes the demonstration or information clear and interesting/exciting, it is more likely that the performer will remember that information.

The rehearsal loop – this is the mental rehearsal of actions found in the short-term memory shown in Atkinson's model in Figure 4.1.1; for example, when the netball player is mentally rehearsing her coach's instructions.

The visuo-spatial sketchpad – this allows the temporary holding of a visual image. The process stores and processes information in a visual or spatial form via a visualisation technique that can be practised by the sports performer. For example, the netball player will visualise a particular attacking move and this move is then stored as a visual representation in the visuo-spatial sketchpad.

The executive control system – this controls the limited amount of information that may be judged at any one time, as the performer make decisions. The player may weigh up two or three possible moves before selecting the one she feels will be the most successful.

IN THE NEWS

VISUALISING TO HELP MEMORY AND TO FOCUS

Chris Smalling has revealed he spends four hours a month visiting a sports psychologist to ensure he is ready for matches with Manchester United. He revealed in an interview with the *Daily Telegraph* that he visits a psychologist twice a month for a couple of hours at a time, to help him to prepare mentally for the pressures of playing for the club. During the sessions, he uses visualisation to focus his mind on upcoming matches, and to 'unclutter' his mind and focus on what is important.

You can read the full article from the *Daily Telegraph* on 5 December 2013, at: www.telegraph.co.uk/sport/football/teams/manchester-united/12034908/Man-Utd-news-Chris-Smalling-reveals-he-visits-sports-psychologist-twice-a-month.html

Another view of memory

Both the STM (short-term memory) and the LTM (long-term memory) are used by the table tennis player in perception and making decisions. To hit the ball there is constant referral to what is already known (LTM) and what is about to happen (STM). Baddeley (1986) called the STM the 'working memory' because of this information going back and forth from and to the LTM. According to Baddeley, there are three components of the working memory: the central executive, the phonological loop and the visuo-spatial sketchpad.

Source: Baddeley, A. (1986) *Working Memory*. Oxford: Oxford University Press

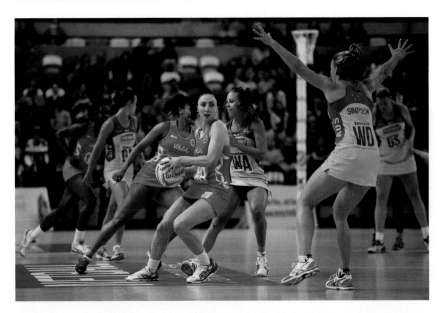

▲ Figure 4.1.3 The netball player will visualise a particular attacking move that will help to store a visual image in the visuo-spatial sketchpad

Relating both models to the learning and performance of physical activity skills

To make our memory processes more effective so that we can optimise learning and sports performance, there are a number of ways in which memory can be improved:

● Rehearsal – this can be useful for retrieval of information in both the short-term memory and the long-term memory, as shown in the multi-store memory model.

  ● Practical example: the tennis player will rehearse her serve physically as well as mentally by practising the throw-up of the ball, the preparation backswing, the strike and the follow-through.

● Meaningfulness – the more the information is seen as relevant to our needs, the more likely we are to remember it, as shown in the levels of processing model.

  ● Practical example: the tennis coach will show that the coaching information being given will raise the player's performance levels.

- Association – if new information is linked somehow to old information, it is more likely to be remembered, thus associating it with something already known, especially relevant to the levels of processing approach.
  - Practical example: the tennis coach will show the player that new information regarding the serve technique is simply an adaptation of the old serve, so the learning of a whole new skill is not required.
- Avoiding overload – any new information must be allowed to 'sink in', thus avoiding potential confusion, relating particularly to the multi-store memory model.
  - Practical example: the tennis coach will give only a few points for the player to remember before the match.
- Organise information – we have seen that chunking can expand the STM store. Complex pieces of information should be grouped to aid understanding, relevant to the multi-store memory model.
  - Practical example: the trampolinist will remember a complex sequence by mentally putting together the small moves to make bigger ones.

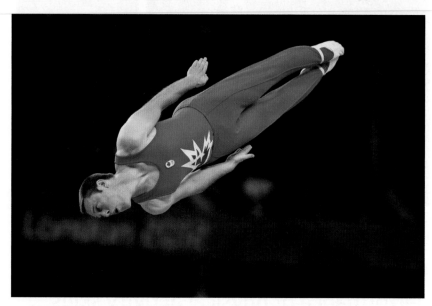

▲ Figure 4.1.4 A trampolinist will use chunking to remember a sequence

- Mental imagery – a performer will often remember a visual representation far more than verbal instructions. This is especially relevant to the levels of processing approach.
  - Practical example: the trampoline coach demonstrates the move to the performer or shows him a video of the sequence so that he can remember it more effectively.

Summary

- There are three stages of remembering information according to the multi-store memory approach: encoding, storage, retrieval.
- The basic model describes memory as essentially a three-stage process: short-term sensory store → short-term memory → long-term memory.
- In selective attention, relevant information is filtered through into the short-term memory and irrelevant information is lost or forgotten.
- Chunking is a process of organising information to improve the effectiveness of the short-term memory.
- The levels of processing model seeks to explain what we do with the information rather than how it is stored. How deeply we consider or process information dictates how long the memory lasts.
- How much this information is considered is called the 'depth of processing'. The deeper the information is processed, the longer the memory or memory trace will last.
- The application of the levels of processing approach to learning movement skills necessitates that instructions and demonstrations be able to show or elicit meaning from the activity.
- Research has revealed that other aspects of how information is given or presented can affect how deep a performer's processing might be.
- Rehearsal, meaningfulness and association are the three ways in which memory can be enhanced.

Check your understanding

1. What are the main elements of Atkinson and Shiffren's multi-store memory model?
2. What practical example would you use to explain the multi-store memory model?
3. What is the purpose of selective attention?
4. What are the main features of Craik and Lockhart's levels of processing model?
5. What practical example would you use to explain the levels of processing model?
6. How do both models relate to the learning and performance of physical activity skills?

Practice questions

1 Draw the multi-store memory model and outline how it seeks to explain the learning of a selected movement skill in sport. (6 marks)

2 Using a practical example from learning a sports skill, explain what is meant by selective attention. (3 marks)

3 Explain the main features of the levels of processing model of memory. (5 marks)

4 Using one practical example, explain how we remember how to perform a physical activity skill according to the levels of processing model of memory. (10 marks)

5 Explain the relationship between memory and personal relevance when learning physical activity skills. (5 marks)

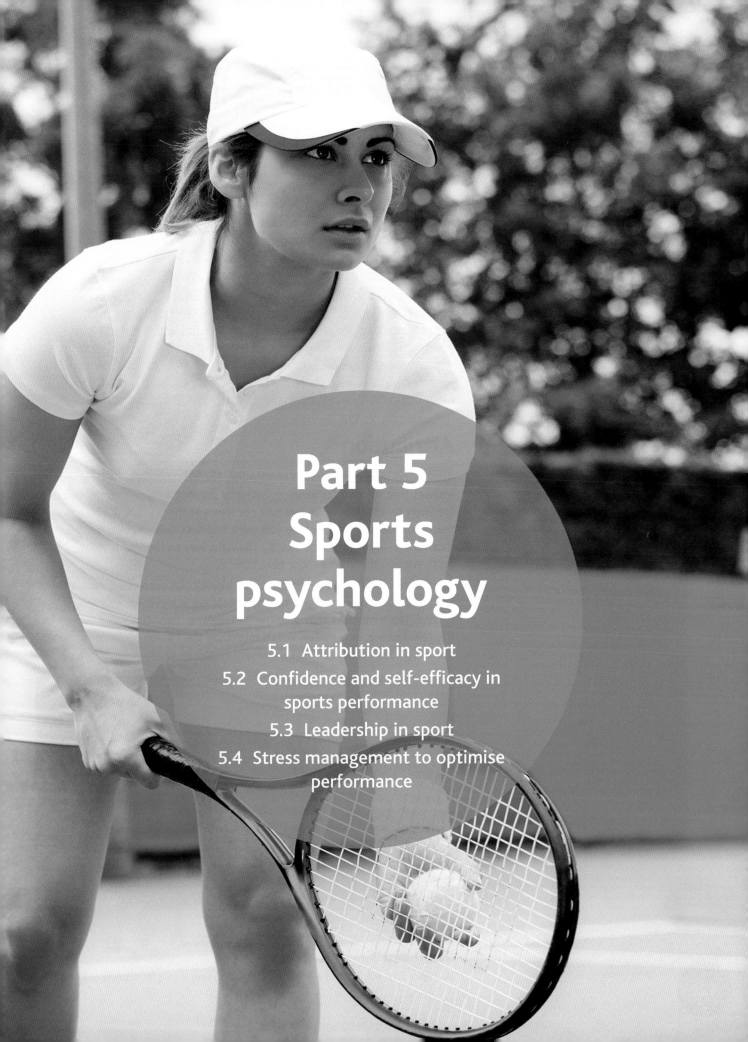

Part 5
Sports psychology

5.1 Attribution in sport
5.2 Confidence and self-efficacy in sports performance
5.3 Leadership in sport
5.4 Stress management to optimise performance

5.1 Attribution in sport

Understanding the specification

By the end of this chapter you should:

- be able to describe and explain Weiner's model of attribution, including the dimensions of stability, locus of control and controllability
- have developed an understanding of learned helplessness as a barrier to sports performance and about mastery orientation to optimise sports performance.

The introduction to sports psychology in Book 1 followed the influences of individual differences that affect behaviour in sport, such as personality and attitudes. In Book 2 we explore in more detail psychological aspects that impact directly on sports performance, such as levels of confidence, influences of leadership and stress. In this chapter we consider attribution as a key concept that can motivate or demotivate sports performers.

Attribution

Attribution theory is linked to motivation. The reasons, justifications and excuses that we give for winning, losing or drawing in sports competitions are likely to affect how we feel and our levels of motivation. If a coach tells you that you lost because you were hopeless, this might lower your motivation – or it might be exactly the right way to fire you up and motivate you to achieve more next time.

Attributions are the perceived causes of a particular outcome. In sport these are often the reasons we give for the results we achieve. For example, a football team member may give the bad weather conditions as a reason for the team losing, or a netball coach might say the reason for winning was the team's high level of effort.

Activity

Think back to your last competitive experience in a sports activity. Write down the reasons that you can think of now for the result you achieved.

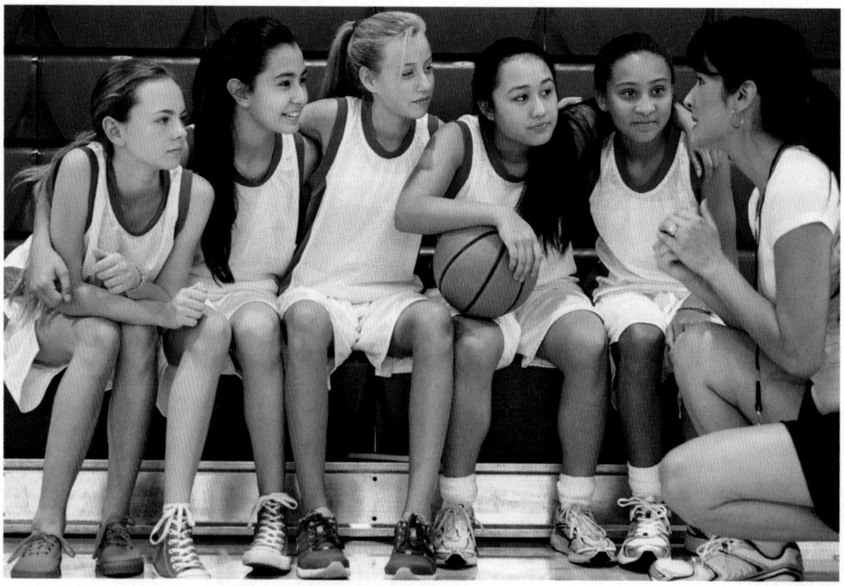

▲ Figure 5.1.1 Attributions are reasons that sports people give for winning or losing

122

Attributions are important because of the way in which they affect motivation, which in turn affects future performances, future effort and even whether the individual continues to participate in sport.

A young person who is told that they failed because they do not have enough ability to succeed is unlikely to try again. If the same individual is given reasons that he can work on, such as 'need to put in more effort', he is more likely to continue and to heed the advice.

The model in Figure 5.1.2 is a well-known representation of the process of attribution. At times, inappropriate or unreal attributions are given, but for the sake of future success, it is important to change these to ones that are going to be far more helpful and more motivating. This is known as attribution retraining.

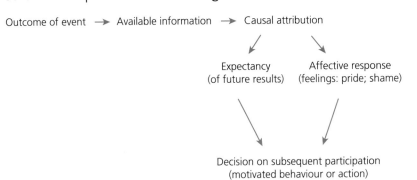

Outcome of event → Available information → Causal attribution

Expectancy (of future results)   Affective response (feelings: pride; shame)

Decision on subsequent participation (motivated behaviour or action)

▲ Figure 5.1.2 The process of attribution

Weiner's model of attribution

Weiner (1979) identified four main reasons given for examination results: ability, effort, task difficulty and luck. He then constructed a two-dimensional model, which he called the locus of causality and stability.

The locus of causality refers to whether the attributions come from within the person (internal) or from the environment (external) and affects a person's feelings of pride, confidence and shame.

Stability refers to whether the attribution is changeable or unchangeable and affects a person's expectations of future outcomes. Weiner's classification for causal attributions is shown in Figure 5.1.3.

Locus of causality

	Internal	External
Stable	Ability (internal/stable)	Task difficulty (external/stable)
Unstable	Effort (internal/unstable)	Luck (external/unstable)

Stability dimension

▲ Figure 5.1.3 Weiner's model of attribution

Weiner's model is not sports specific, which causes problems when trying to apply it to sports situations. For instance, task difficulty changes frequently in sport, especially in team games, because the opposition changes. This model can be applied to sport in a general sense, however, and can be used to promote reasons for sports outcomes that can be motivating rather than demotivating.

If the reasons given for winning are stable, the individual is motivated to achieve again. If failure is attributed to an unstable factor, the individual is more likely to try again because there is a good chance that the outcome will change.

RESEARCH IN FOCUS

Roberts and Pascuzzi (1979) related Weiner's model to sport. They found that the two-dimensional model was still relevant, but that far more attributions were given than Weiner's main four. Their model is shown in Figure 5.1.4.

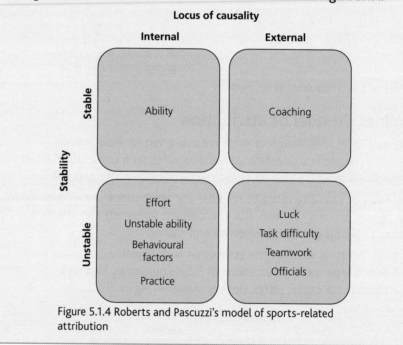

Figure 5.1.4 Roberts and Pascuzzi's model of sports-related attribution

Sports performers who lose tend to attribute their failure to external causes, while those who succeed usually attribute their success to internal causes. This is known as the **self-serving bias**.

IN THE NEWS

A newspaper article illustrates the types of attributions given by football managers that are also examples of self-serving bias – for example, disputed decisions by the referee or his assistant. Instead of giving external reasons for defeat, the article calls for managers to take a step back and look at their own players' mistakes instead, such as a striker fluffing a sitter, or a defender mis-kicking a back pass which ultimately leads to the opposition scoring.

You can read the full article from the *Daily Mirror* on 25 October 2015, at www.mirror.co.uk/sport/football/news/its-time-premier-league-managers-6700505

Controllability

Weiner added a third dimension to his attribution model – the dimension of **controllability**, which he thought reflected the view that we have greater or lesser personal control over event outcomes.

This dimension takes into consideration whether a cause for a sports outcome is controllable or uncontrollable. Figure 5.1.5 shows how controllability is affected by each type of attribution.

Coaches and teachers tend to praise effort and controllable success, and punish or criticise lack of effort and controllable failures. Concentrating on uncontrollable external and stable factors is not of much use if you want to turn failure into success.

Key term

Controllability: whether attributions are under the control of the performer or under the control of others, or whether they are uncontrollable (i.e. nothing can be done by anyone, e.g. luck, weather).

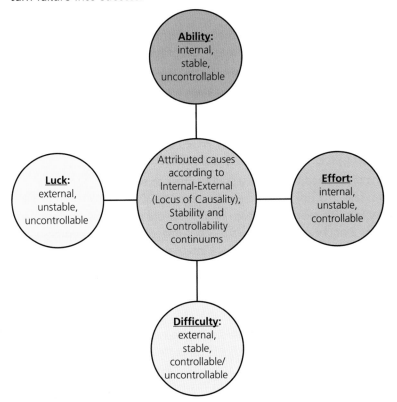

▲ Figure 5.1.5 Attribution theory: how each attributed cause links to controllability

Learned helplessness

This refers to a belief that failure is inevitable and a feeling of hopelessness when faced with a particular situation (specific learned helplessness) or groups of situations (global learned helplessness). For example:

- Specific learned helplessness: 'I am a hopeless football player.'
- Global learned helplessness: 'I am hopeless at all sport.'

Low achievers often attribute their failure to uncontrollable factors, which can lead to learned helplessness. High achievers are athletes who are oriented towards mastery and see failure as a learning experience, and who will attribute failure to controllable unstable factors. The 'need to achieve' (Nach) performers are not afraid of failing and will persist with a task until they succeed.

Mastery orientation

Mastery orientation is the view that an individual will be motivated by becoming an expert (master) in skill development or sports performance. An athlete who is mastery orientated will often attribute failure to internal, controllable and unstable factors, such as effort, and will continue to strive to become better at the activity. They seek to develop their competence by acquiring new skills and mastering new situations. They are not concerned about their performance relative to others, but rather with furthering their understanding of their sport, fitness and sport performance. Mastery orientation is at the opposite end of the scale to learned helplessness, which is the belief that failure is inevitable and that the individual has no control over the factors that cause failure.

Attribution retraining

Attribution retraining can optimise sports performance – seeking often to change learned helplessness into mastery orientation.

Many attributions that are given are subjective and are therefore not desirable for future progression. For instance, a hockey player used to play for a team that constantly blamed the officials for their poor results. Although this helped to draw the team together, the team had a bad reputation with most officials and they were not attributing their poor results to changeable or (in this case) realistic factors.

Attributions often need to be reassessed in order to succeed in the future. A person who fails in a task should be encouraged to attribute to controllable, unstable factors. For example, a team of 17-year-old girls who have just narrowly lost a hockey match should be encouraged to give attributions such as 'must try harder next week' (these are internal, unstable and controllable). Using attribution in this way is more likely to result in mastery orientation.

Evaluation

To help those who have failed and are starting to experience learned helplessness, teachers and coaches should concentrate on the positive attributions. If a performer feels that they lack ability, they will inevitably fail, but their attribution could be changed to 'having the wrong tactics' or 'slight alteration of technique needed'. The performer may then be disappointed rather than frustrated and will persist with the task rather than avoid it altogether. This process is known as attribution retraining.

Summary

- Attributions are the reasons we give for winning or losing and can affect motivation and therefore future performance.
- Weiner's model of attribution is two-dimensional, including where the attributions have come from (the locus of causality) and whether they are stable or not (the locus of stability). A third dimension (controllability) has been added, which refers to whether the performer has control over the causes of failure.
- Low achievers can suffer from learned helplessness, which can be global or specific.
- Attributing to uncontrollable, stable and internal factors can lead to learned helplessness.
- An athlete who is mastery orientated will often attribute failure to internal factors, such as effort, and will continue to strive to become better at the activity.
- Attribution retraining can help to change attributions and minimise the effects of learned helplessness.

Check your understanding

1 What is meant by the attribution process?
2 What does the stability dimension show in Weiner's attribution model?
3 What is meant by controllability when applied to attribution?
4 How does the locus of control affect controllability?
5 Why is learned helplessness a barrier to sports performance?
6 How does mastery orientation lead to high-level performance?

Practice questions

1 Explain Weiner's model of attribution using examples from sport. (8 marks)

2 As a coach, justify the types of attributions you might encourage your team to give following a lost match. (6 marks)

3 What is meant by learned helplessness in sports performance? (4 marks)

4 Using attributional theory and practical examples, explain how learned helplessness experienced by an athlete might be modified into mastery orientation. (10 marks)

5.2 Confidence and self-efficacy in sports performance

Understanding the specification

By the end of this chapter you should be able to:

- define key terms related to sports confidence and self-efficacy
- understand the impact of sports confidence on performance, participation and self-esteem
- understand Vealey's model of sports confidence and Bandura's theory of self-efficacy and be able to explain these using practical examples from sport.

Key terms

Sports confidence: the belief or degree of certainty individuals possess about their ability to be successful in sport.

Self-efficacy: the self-confidence we have in specific situations.

Study hint

Learn definitions along with practical examples for sports confidence and self-efficacy. Be able to give sports examples for both.

Activity

Write down the situations in your sport where you feel a low sense of self-efficacy. How do you account for these feelings of low self-efficacy?

If you were to coach a young girl in the high jump and she initially had low levels of self-efficacy, how would you raise her self-efficacy to make her more motivated to succeed?

Key term

Self-esteem: the feeling of self-worth that determines how valuable and competent we feel.

Motivation is often affected by the degree of self-confidence that an individual possesses. **Sports confidence** is a rather global term, which infers a general disposition or feeling we may have in a variety of situations in sport. Having high levels of sports confidence is often associated with someone having little doubt that they will achieve in sport or, for example, be accepted in a sports team. When you have high levels of sports confidence, you have a firm belief in your own judgements and ability in sport. The term **self-efficacy** is often used for self-confidence in a specific situation. A person who has belief in their ability to achieve success will have high self-efficacy – for example, a tennis player's belief in how many first serves will be successful.

Our expectations of whether or not sports confidence is going to be high or low may determine the activity we choose, the amount of effort we put into it and whether we stick with the task or give up easily.

Sports performance, participation and self-esteem

Sports confidence can have an impact on sports performance because you may be more motivated to achieve and will take firm decisions that are more likely to have positive outcomes in sport if you have high self-confidence. For example, an athlete with high levels of sports confidence in the 100 m sprint is more likely to achieve a better time than someone with low sports confidence.

Sports confidence can have an impact on participation. Those who have low sports confidence may shy away from activities and avoid situations that may be related to competition, for instance. High sports confidence would enable them to participate with other people and not feel inhibited, and feel more able to engage in team activities.

Sports confidence can affect levels of **self-esteem**. Those with high levels of sports confidence will often have high self-esteem, which will help performance because sport often demands high levels of arousal or drive to achieve. Those with low levels of sports confidence may experience low self-esteem and feel that they are not good enough or valuable enough to contribute to team or individual sports performance.

IN THE NEWS

The former British National Mountain Bike champion Lee Craigie reports the benefits of sport for self-esteem and confidence. Lee is a fully trained child and adolescent psychotherapist as well as an accomplished mountain biker. Her project 'Cycletherapy' is aimed at socially excluded young people in the Scottish Highlands whose needs are not met in mainstream education. The programme benefits young people's self-esteem through teaching mountain biking and bike repair skills.

From an early age, sports experiences can positively or negatively affect a child's self-esteem. Relationships with parents, coaches and team mates can all have an impact. Problems with self-esteem can continue into later life if they are not addressed.

Positive self-esteem is key to psychological well-being. Children with positive self-esteem are better able to cope with wins and losses in sports and in life.

These enhanced coping skills can translate into lifetime benefits, such as:

- reduced anxiety
- a more optimistic outlook on life
- fewer interpersonal problems
- less chance of conforming to social pressure
- better body image
- being less likely to engage in risky behaviours, such as drug use.

Children with negative self-esteem are more likely to:

- be depressed
- have eating disorders
- engage in risky behaviours
- not participate in sports or physical activity
- get bullied or become bullies.

Self-esteem can be enhanced by positive experiences in sports.

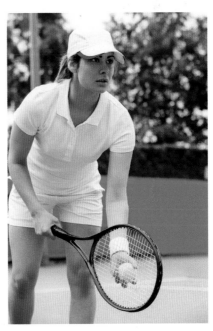

▲ Figure 5.2.1 Sports confidence can affect performance in sport

Vealey's sport confidence model

Vealey's sport-specific model of sport confidence (1986) investigates the relationship between achievement motivation or competitiveness and self-confidence in sport. The model shown in Figure 5.2.2 is situation-specific and shows that sport confidence can be affected by a number of factors.

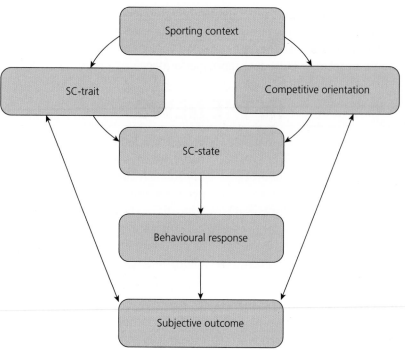

▲ Figure 5.2.2 Vealey's sport confidence model

Vealey's model shows that every sports person or athlete has an existing level of sport confidence, which is a trait (SC-trait), and an existing level of competitiveness (competitive orientation). The amounts of SC-trait and competitive orientation are indicative of the confidence that can be shown in a specific situation in sport (SC-state) or level of self-efficacy during competition. (See Book 1, Part 5.1 on trait and state personality.) According to this model, the level of SC-state then dictates the behaviour that is shown and the skill level of the performance. If the athlete has a high level of SC-state, their behaviour is more likely to be confident and well motivated, and consequently performance is likely to improve. If, however, SC-state is low, then the athlete's behaviour is likely to be tentative and lacking in confidence, and they may therefore turn in a poor performance.

After the performance, either satisfaction or disappointment will prevail. These emotions, known as the **subjective perceptions of outcome**, will in turn affect the athlete's confidence and competitiveness in future performances. Simply put, the more confident you are, the more successful you will be, and the more successful you are, the more confident you will be.

Young athletes should be helped to gain confidence in at least one sport or activity. This will enhance the general perception of sport confidence because the more sports they experience, the more likely they are to be successful. As the young athlete's personality traits develop, they will experience greater levels of situation-specific sport confidence with new sports and activities. These young people will then be much more likely to be motivated to persist in sports activities.

Key term

Subjective perceptions of outcome: how someone interprets their performance in sport.

Bandura's theory of self-efficacy

According to Bandura (1977), self-confidence can often be specific to a particular situation. Bandura called this self-efficacy. This specific confidence can vary from situation to situation and, according to Bandura, can affect performance if the individual is skilful enough. People who expect to be confident in a particular situation are more likely to choose that activity. Conversely, people who expect to have low self-efficacy in a situation will avoid that particular activity.

Our expectations of self-efficacy depend on four types of information, according to Bandura's theory of self-efficacy (1977):

1   Performance accomplishments. These probably have the strongest influence on self-confidence. If success has been experienced in the past, especially if it has been attributed to controllable factors, then feelings of self-confidence are likely to be high.

2   Vicarious experiences. These refer to what we have observed before. If we watch others perform and be successful, then we are more likely to experience high self-efficacy, as long as the performers we are watching are of a similar standard.

3   Verbal persuasion. If we are encouraged to try a particular activity, our confidence in that situation may increase. The effectiveness of this encouragement depends upon who is encouraging us and in what ways. Significant others (for instance, friends and family) are more likely to persuade us to 'have a go' than strangers.

4   Emotional arousal. Our perceptions of how aroused we are can affect our confidence in a particular situation. If you have effective strategies to control physiological and psychological arousal levels (perhaps the ability to relax or to use mental rehearsal), you are more likely to have high self-efficacy.

These factors are illustrated in Figure 5.2.3.

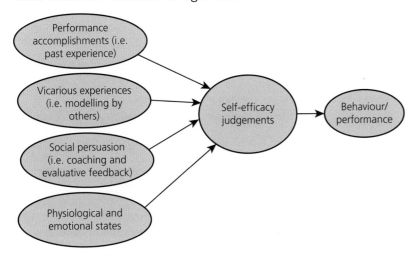

▲ Figure 5.2.3 Bandura's model of self-efficacy showing sources of efficacy information in sport

RESEARCH IN FOCUS
Raising self-efficacy in sport

Here are a few strategies that you could use to raise the level of self-efficacy of the athlete featured in the activity at the start of this chapter who has low self-efficacy in the high jump.

1   Try to give her initial success by lowering the bar to start with, or using some flexi-rope.

2   Demonstrate how it can be done or, if you are much better than her, use someone of similar ability. An actual demonstration (live modelling) can be more effective than a video recording in raising self-confidence.

3   Verbally encourage the athlete. Tell her that she should 'have a go', that she will succeed – even that the mat is nice and soft!

4   Tell her that to be worried is a natural, very positive response because it prepares the body well. Alternatively, teach her some relaxation techniques or how to mentally rehearse the activity (but be aware that this could increase her anxiety).

Source: Bandura (1977)

Summary

- Sports confidence is the belief or degree of certainty individuals possess about their ability to be successful in sport.
- Sports confidence can affect performance, participation and self-esteem.
- Self-efficacy is self-confidence in a specific situation.
- Vealey's sport-specific model of sport confidence investigates the relationship between achievement motivation or competitiveness and self-confidence in sport.
- According to Vealey, the more confident you are, the more successful you will be, and the more successful you are, the more confident you will be.
- Expectations of self-efficacy are closely linked to motivation and can affect the choice of activity, the amount of effort expended and persistence at the task.
- Bandura's factors affecting expectations are performance accomplishments, vicarious experiences, verbal persuasion and emotional arousal.

Check your understanding

1   What is meant by sports confidence and self-efficacy in sport?

2   How does sports confidence affect performance, participation and self-esteem?

3   What does Vealey's model of sports confidence show?

4   What are the four factors that affect self-efficacy according to Bandura?

Practice questions

1   What are the definitions of sports confidence and
    self-efficacy?   (2 marks)

2   Using practical examples, explain how sports confidence
    impacts on performance, participation and self-esteem.   (5 marks)

3   Using a practical example, describe how each stage of
    Bandura's self-efficacy model can have an effect on
    performance in sport.   (6 marks)

4   Describe what is meant by sports confidence. Explain
    how you might increase the level of sports confidence by using
    Vealey's model of sports confidence.   (10 marks)

5.3 Leadership in sport

Understanding the specification

By the end of this chapter you should:

- know the characteristics of effective leaders in sport and be able to describe emergent and prescribed leaders
- have an understanding about autocratic, democratic and laissez-faire leadership styles and give practical examples
- be familiar with the trait perspective, social learning and interactionist theories of leadership
- have an understanding of Chelladurai's multi-dimensional model of sports leadership and be able to explain it using practical examples.

Leadership

Leadership in sport can be defined as an individual having enough influence over the behaviour of others to motivate them to follow the individual's own set goals. Effective leadership can affect performance of individuals and teams in all sports. A good leader can motivate others and can give focus or direction to attaining goals such as success and enjoyment in sport.

There are many leader positions in sport, for example:

- captain
- manager
- director
- coach
- physiotherapist
- team sports psychologist.

Leadership is important in influencing behaviour in sport. Team captains, managers, coaches and teachers all need leadership qualities. Sports psychologist Barrow (1977) saw leadership as 'the behavioural process influencing individuals and groups towards set goals'. The key words in this definition are 'influencing' and 'set goals'. Leadership involves personal relationships and affects the motivation of individuals and groups.

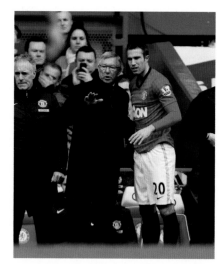

▲ Figure 5.3.1 Good leadership in sport can affect motivation and performance

Effective leadership

An effective leader has a number of qualities; no single quality will ensure effectiveness on its own. Qualities of leadership include:

- good communication skills
- high motivation
- enthusiasm

- having a clear goal or a vision of what needs to be achieved
- empathy (an ability to put yourself in the position of others to understand how they feel)
- being good at the sport themselves or having a comprehensive knowledge of the sport
- charisma – this is a quality that is difficult to analyse, but the person who has charisma is hard to ignore, and has a certain 'presence' and great powers of persuasion.

Some of these qualities may be learned, some may be seen as innate or natural – it is commonly thought that a leader is born, not made.

Emergent and prescribed leaders

Emergent leaders come from within the group because they are skilful or because the rest of the team selected them. Prescribed leaders are appointed to a team from an external source. There are advantages and disadvantages in both methods of becoming a leader.

Emergent leaders can win over the 'hearts and minds' of team mates because they are recognised as being one of their own, rather than an unknown and potentially threatening 'outsider'. The disadvantage here is that an emergent leader may lack objectivity and have their own friendships within the group that might colour their judgements; for example, for a captain or manager making team selection decisions.

Prescribed leaders have the advantage of being more objective and could bring to a team or individuals a 'fresh pair of eyes', which might result in more creative strategies being implemented. Prescribed leaders may carry more authority or power that has been given to them by others. The disadvantage of a prescribed leader might be that they do not share or are not aware of the team culture or ways of working or friendship groups, and this might delay effective decision-making.

Leadership styles

Many different styles of leadership have been identified. It is generally agreed that leadership can be divided into three styles:

1 Autocratic or authoritarian leaders are task oriented and are more dictatorial in style. They make most of the decisions and tend to have commanding and directing approaches. They show little interest in the individuals making up the group.

2 Democratic leaders are person oriented and value the views of other group members. These leaders tend to share decisions and show a good deal of interest in the individuals of the group.

3 Laissez-faire leaders make very few decisions and give very little feedback. The individual group members mostly do as they wish.

Activity

Construct a table outlining the advantages and disadvantages of an emergent leader and a prescribed leader. Reflect on your own experiences and state which situations would suit which type of leader.

Summary of each leadership style and when they are best used in sports situations

Autocratic style

Description	When the leader makes most of the decisions and concentrates on the job to be done or is more concerned with the end product, such as performance or winning, or has a clear, pre-determined goal.
Explanation of use	Used when discipline and control are needed or when there are hostile groups involved. Used also if there is a lack of time or for the early stage (cognitive stage) of learning. Novice performers, team players and males are generally found to prefer an autocratic leadership style from their leader. If a situation is dangerous, or when the task is clear and unambiguous, this style is best. Also if the leader's personality is autocratic or authoritarian.

Democratic style

Description	This is when the leader is more concerned with interpersonal relations and is more person/social orientated in their approach. This leader invites contributions and shares the decision-making.
Explanation of use	When group members wish or are able to participate in decision-making and for those who prefer this democratic approach. This style suits more advanced performers who have the knowledge to contribute or to motivate group members. A social or 'friendly' match suits this style, or when a task demands greater interpersonal communication and if the leader and group members are well known to each other. Some research has shown that females are more likely to prefer this democratic or social approach. If the task or situation is not dangerous, this style is suitable. This democratic style is also suited to small teams or for individual sports people. This style is suitable if the leader's personality lends itself to a democratic or social approach or when there is more time available.

Laissez-faire style

Description	This is when the leader has no direct influence on group members or the leader takes a back seat and lets the group members make their own decisions.
Explanation of use	This is suitable for high-level performers or elite athletes. This style helps to develop creativity for team members or individuals and the leader has full trust in members' capabilities. This style is suitable if the task involves individual decision-making or if the leader is creating an assessment situation or assessing the group members. This style may also be adopted if the leader is incompetent or is unable to employ any other style of leadership.

Coaches and teachers should not rely too heavily on the autocratic approach – it may result in hostility and may deter athletes from taking on any personal responsibility in situations where their coach isn't present. The democratic approach may result in less work being done but will increase the positive effects of interaction. The laissez-faire approach should be actively avoided in most situations, although this style does encourage more creativity among team members and also gives them more responsibility.

RESEARCH IN FOCUS

The eminent psychologist Lewin (1939) led an historical piece of research that is still relevant today. Lewin looked at the styles of leadership that group members preferred. He studied a group of ten-year-old boys attending after-school clubs which were led by adults using the three different styles. Boys with an autocratic leader became aggressive towards each other when things went wrong and were submissive in their approach to the leader. If the leader left the room, they stopped working. Boys with a democratic leader got on with each other much better. They did slightly less work than the group with an autocratic leader, but their work was comparable in quality. When the teacher left the room, the boys carried on working. With the laissez-faire leader, the boys were aggressive towards each other, did very little work and were easily discouraged.

Quite a lot of research has been undertaken on the styles of leader that group members prefer. A good leader will not shy away from making unpopular decisions but should consider the preferences of the group when making decisions. Sports psychologist Chelladurai led research to determine whether certain leadership theories were applicable to the sporting environment. He listed five dimensions of leadership.

1 Training and instruction behaviour improves performance and emphasises hard training – it is a very structured approach.

2 Democratic behaviour – allows group participation in decision-making.

3 Autocratic behaviour – the coach makes the decisions and stresses their personal authority.

4 Social support behaviour – the coach has concern for individuals and there is a positive and warm atmosphere in the team.

5 Rewarding behaviour – recognises and reinforces good performances.

Activity

Identify your preferences for coaching behaviour, either as a coach or as a performer. What sort of atmosphere do you thrive in?

Your response to the last activity will probably depend on who you are coaching or being coached by and the situation you are in. Some generalisations may be made from the available research findings.

The results of research by sports psychologists led by Crust (2006) in a review of leadership in sport show the following:

1 Novice athletes prefer more rewards and experts prefer more democratic and social support coaching.

2 Team members prefer more training and instruction, autocratic coaching and rewards. Individual sports people prefer democratic coaching and social support.

3 Male athletes prefer a more autocratic style of coaching and females prefer a democratic style.

4 Older athletes prefer democratic coaching, social support and training and instruction. Athletes of all ages seem to value rewards equally.

A 'CONFRONTATIONAL' LEADERSHIP STYLE OF PREMIER LEAGUE MANAGER

In an article in *The Guardian* in March 2015, José Mourinho, manager of Chelsea FC at the time, provided an insight into his man-management tricks, such as criticising players in public to motivate them. Mourinho said that his squad might have benefited from 'confrontational leadership', even if he wondered whether many of them could have handled it. Mourinho described confrontational leadership as being 'when you are ready to provoke your players, to try to create some conflict, with the intention to bring out the best from them'. You can read the full article on *The Guardian* website at: www.theguardian.com/football/2015/mar/20/chelsea-jose-mourinho.

Activity

Which style of leadership would you adopt in the following situations?
- You are introducing yourself as the new coach to a hostile group.
- You would like to bring together a very large group of athletes as a team before a big meeting.
- You are coaching a highly skilled squash player.
- A friendly, successful team of lacrosse players ask you to be their coach.
- A novice weightlifter needs coaching just before the lift.

Give reasons for your answers. (You should take into consideration the three main influences: characteristic of the leader, situational factors, team members' characteristics.)

Theories of leadership

Having looked at the styles of leadership, it is important to explore how people become leaders in sport. We will look specifically at the trait perspective, social learning theory and the interactionist approach. These theories can also be applied to many aspects of sports psychology (see, for example, Book 1, page 184, on personality in sport).

Study hint

These theories have been covered before under personality – link the main points and learn evaluation points that are applicable to both personality and leadership topics.

Trait perspective

This view of leadership claims that leaders have a genetic disposition or innate characteristics that show leader qualities, thus lending support to the popular belief that 'great leaders are born and not made'. It is widely agreed that leaders do have certain characteristics that make them effective, but there is some doubt as to whether this is wholly down to an innate disposition. The trait perspective shows that leadership traits are stable and enduring and can be generalised across different situations that make some people leaders in whatever situation they find themselves in. The argument against this theory is that people in sport tend to be quite specific in their leadership skills, depending on their particular situation, which works against the more generalised approach of the trait perspective.

So the trait perspective assumes that:

- certain traits produce certain patterns of behaviour
- these patterns are consistent across different situations
- people are born with these leadership traits.

RESEARCH IN FOCUS
Is a leader born or made?

The early instinct theory related to leadership has been called the Great Man theory. This theory was popularised by the historian Thomas Carlyle in the nineteenth century. It states that leaders are usually male and are born to lead because they have certain personality traits. It ignores situational factors, interactions with others and, of course, that females also make good leaders, so this view on its own has little value. It is, however, still quite a popular view outside sports psychology research.

Social learning theory

As we have explored in the chapter on personality (see Book 1, Chapter 5.1), social learning can be a strong influence on behaviour. This theory claims that leadership characteristics are learned from others. Behaviour of others is watched and copied – we call this **vicarious learning** or vicarious reinforcement.

If you observe another (the model) showing leadership behaviour and that person is of higher status than you, then you are more likely to copy that behaviour. We refer to the model in this case as a role model or a 'significant other'. (See Book 1, Chapter 5.1 on personality for more information.)

According to social learning theory a person in sport, whether it is a coach or a player, may show leadership behaviour that has been learned from other significant people. This theory shows the importance of the social environment for adopting leadership qualities, rather than the trait approach, which does not take the environment into account.

Interactionist theory

We have, again, looked at this in detail in Book 1 in Chapter 5.1 related to personality. The same theory applies with the learning of leadership characteristics. This theory states that an individual may well have certain in-born traits, such as assertiveness, but they are not evident unless a situation (state) demands the leadership behaviour. This theory accounts for the fact that some people are not generally leaders in everyday life, but they can show leadership qualities in sports situations. The interactionist approach involves the interaction of traits (innate) and the changing environment.

Evaluation

More recent research has focused on a **contingency approach** to leadership, which proposes that people in sport who possess certain traits can be more effective in some leadership situations and less so in others. Therefore, leadership qualities might be seen in situations of high anxiety when a team is losing – for example, in a football cup final – or they might arise in situations that require democratic decision-making – for example, involving the team in making decisions on the field of play. One of the major criticisms of trait theory is its simplistic approach and that it fails to take account of other factors that will influence the development of a successful leader – for example, situational and environmental factors.

Key term

Contingency approach: the success of leadership traits is determined by situational factors.

Key term

Vicarious learning: the person observes that a reward is given to another person for certain behaviours and learns to emulate that same behaviour.

Fiedler's contingency model of leadership

Fiedler (1967) proposed a model which looked at the way the leader interacts with the situation they find themselves in. He used two classifications of leader – the task-oriented leader (focus on performance) and the person-oriented leader (focus on personal relationships). He saw that the effectiveness of these leaders depends on the favourableness of the situation, which itself depends on:

- the relationship between the leader and the group members
- the structure of the task
- the leader's power and position of authority.

The situation is most favourable if the relationships between leader and group members are warm and positive, the task is clear and unambiguous, and the leader is in a strong position of authority. If a situation is unfavourable, the opposites apply.

According to Fiedler, task-oriented leaders are more effective in situations that are at the extremes (most favourable or least favourable). Person-oriented leaders are most effective in situations that are moderately favourable.

Chelladurai's multi-dimensional model of sports leadership

The most popular view of leadership is that people learn to be leaders through social learning and interactions with their environment. Chelladurai's multi-dimensional model of leadership (1984), shown in Figure 5.3.2, is a popular approach to the study of leadership among sport psychologists.

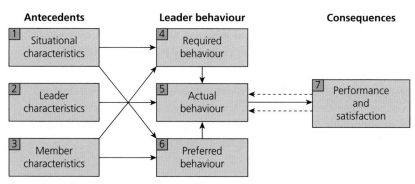

▲ Figure 5.3.2 Chelladurai's multi-dimensional model of leadership

Chelladurai identified three factors or antecedents that affect leadership:

1 The characteristics of the situation (situational characteristics).
2 The characteristics of the leader (leader characteristics).
3 The characteristics of the people who are to be led (member characteristics).

The more the elements of this model match each other, the more effective the leadership is likely to be. If the leadership qualities are what the group want and expect, then they are more likely to follow the leader. If the leadership style matches the situation, again leadership is likely to be more effective. The 'Consequences' in Figure 5.3.2 involve levels of performance of group members (how well they do following leadership intervention) as well as satisfaction (how well they think they have done).

An example of this theory applied to a sports context is as follows:

Antecedents: 1) Situational characteristics: outdoor rock climbing, which is perceived to be dangerous for participants. 2) Leader characteristics: an experienced rock climber. 3) Member characteristics: all group members are novices in rock climbing.

Leader behaviour: 4) Required behaviour: the leader should adopt an autocratic leadership style and give direct instructions to group members because the situation is dangerous and group members are beginners. 6) Preferred behaviour: for the leader to be autocratic, making most of the decisions and telling group members exactly what to do as they are inexperienced. 5) Actual behaviour: the leadership style shown by the leader; in this case, an autocratic approach, giving instructions and making most of the decisions.

Consequences: 7) Performance and satisfaction: the leader's actual behaviour matches the required behaviour and preferred behaviour and so the group show good performance in learning to climb and experience high levels of satisfaction.

The arrows in the model are two-way between points 5 and 7, showing that actual behaviour or leadership style can be modified depending on the performance and satisfaction levels of the group.

Summary

- Leadership involves influencing people towards set goals.
- Leaders can fill positions of responsibility, either by emerging or being prescribed.
- The main styles of leadership are the authoritarian, task-oriented style, the democratic, person-oriented style and the laissez-faire style.
- Most leaders have a mix of styles but tend towards one of them.
- There are preferred styles among sports people, but this depends on situational and group characteristic variables.
- Leaders may be born or made, but research points to social learning or interactionist approaches being most realistic.
- Effective leadership depends on situational factors, the characteristics of the leader, and the expectations and natures of the group members. This is known as the multi-dimensional model of leadership.
- Fiedler's theory states that favourableness of the situation must be considered before adopting a particular style.

Check your understanding

1 What are the main characteristics of effective leaders in sport?
2 What is meant by emerged and prescribed leaders in sport?
3 What are the characteristics of the autocratic, democratic and laissez-faire styles of leadership?
4 In what different situations would you use each of these leadership styles?
5 What are the main features of the trait perspective, social learning theory and interactionist theory of leadership?
6 What does Chelladurai's model of leadership explain about the links between antecedents and leader behaviour?

Practice questions

1 Describe the qualities of an effective leader in sport. (4 marks)
2 Evaluate the effectiveness of leaders who emerge and leaders who are prescribed in sport. (4 marks)
3 Discuss the use of different leadership styles to maximise the performance of a sports team. (10 marks)
4 Explain three main leadership theories using examples from sport. (10 marks)
5 Using the diagram of Chelladurai's multi-dimensional model of leadership, explain how performance and satisfaction are affected by a leader's behaviour. (8 marks)

5.4 Stress management to optimise performance

One of the most important factors separating the very best sportsmen and women from the merely good is the ability to control anxiety at crucial moments in sports events. It is unsurprising, then, that much importance is placed upon managing stress to eliminate anxiety and to optimise performance.

Stress and its causes

An understanding of the concept of **stress** is important if it is to be controlled and channelled in the right direction. A great deal of research highlights the negative influences of stress on health and in sports performance. There are direct links between high levels of stress and numerous diseases, many of them fatal. Fitness of the body and fitness of the mind are important if a performer is to reach the highest level in sport, and for beginners to learn new skills.

This chapter investigates the nature of stress, how and why it occurs, and its links with sporting performance. An important section discusses the management of stress and the many strategies that both performers and coaches can use to limit its negative aspects.

Stress is often associated with the term 'anxiety', although stress can be seen as a positive response that can motivate us or keep us safe.

A sports performer is often referred to as 'stressed' and this may be as a result of their perception that their capabilities may not match the demands imposed upon them.

There is much confusion over the terminology associated with stress. Stress can be extremely beneficial to the sports performer – many people say they thrive under stress, and some participants even seek a stressful situation, which is known as eustress.

Extend your knowledge

Eustress is a type of stress that has a positive effect. The performer actively seeks the thrill of the danger associated with the stressor. A typical activity of this type is bungee jumping.

Key term

Stress: in sport, more often linked to negative feelings and can be seen as a psychological state produced by perceived physiological and psychological forces acting on our sense of well-being.

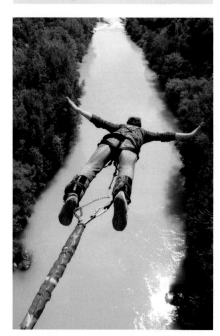

▲ Figure 5.4.1 Sometimes a performer actively seeks the thrill of danger

Physical response to stress

Stress causes a release of hormones in your body. When your body detects stress, a small region in the base of the brain called the hypothalamus reacts by stimulating the body to produce hormones that include adrenaline. These hormones help you to deal with any threats or pressure you are facing, which is called the 'fight or flight' response. Adrenaline increases your heart rate, raises your blood pressure and provides extra energy that is beneficial to sports performance by increasing the amount of oxygen available to the working muscles.

Stress that is too intense or lasts a long time causes your body to release stress hormones over a long period of time. This can increase the risk of a range of health problems, including high blood pressure. It can even increase the risk of having a stroke or heart attack. Stress can also have an extremely negative effect on a performer's readiness to perform and subsequent performance.

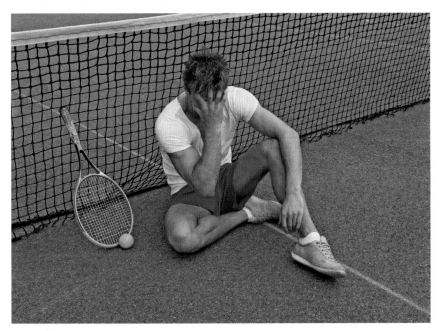

▲ Figure 5.4.2 A performer can be stressed if they perceive that their abilities may not match the demands of the situation

Extend your knowledge

Exercise and stress

Exercise helps to increase the production of endorphins that make us feel good. Endorphins are chemicals called neurotransmitters that transmit electrical signals. Regular exercise can increase levels of self-confidence, improve our mood and lower the risk of depression.

Stressors

The concept of stress can be split into:

- stressors – the environmental changes that can induce a stress response
- stress response – the physiological changes that occur as a result of stress
- stress experience – the way we perceive the situation.

An experience that is potentially stressful is affected by how each of us views that particular experience, and so stress is not inevitable.

A stressor generally arises when there is an imbalance between the person's perception of the demand being made on them by the situation and their ability to meet the demand.

When we experience stress, we often judge how threatening the stressor is and then how able we are to cope with the threat. This concept of coping is important when we investigate stress management techniques.

In sport there are many stressors. However, an experience that is stressful to one person may not be stressful to another.

Competition itself is a powerful stressor. It puts performers into an evaluative position and this can cause apprehension. We will look at competitive anxiety later in this chapter.

Conflict, with other players or the opposition, can be a stressor. A sports person can bring with them social stressors from everyday life, causing conflict within the individual about the choices and decisions that have to be made.

Frustration can also be a stressor. When we investigated aggression in Book 1, Chapter 5.1, we saw that frustration can build up if we are prevented from reaching a goal. Frustration can be caused by our own inadequacies, and by a number of external influences over which we have little control.

Climate can be a stressor. If a sports person has to train in very hot or very cold conditions, this can produce a stressful experience.

In sport the stressor of feeling that you might be physically hurt (not just through injury but through fatigue that hard training or demanding competition often produces) is common.

An example of how different stressors can affect a performer is a golfer who has just reached the third tee and is feeling under stress. The stressors include frustration because he made some poor earlier shots, frustration because he was late due to his car not starting, and frustration because the people in front of him are making slow progress.

Activity

Try to identify what makes you feel under stress in your sport. Do you think that the same stressors will affect someone else in the same way? If not, why not?

Activity

List as many additional stressors as you can that sports people could experience.

Study hint

When considering the causes of stress, refer to different types of stressors and how they might affect a sports performer before, during and after competitive situations. Use practical examples if asked and fully explain each example in terms of why they might be a stressor.

The stress response

The general adaptation syndrome (GAS), devised by the psychologist Selye in 1956, is the most widely accepted theory to explain how our bodies respond to stress. Selye saw GAS as being made up of three stages:

1 The alarm reaction involves physiological changes such as increased heart rate, raised blood sugar levels and adrenaline release.
2 Resistance – if the stressor is not removed, the body begins to recover from the initial alarm reaction and starts to cope with the situation. Adrenaline levels fall.
3 Exhaustion – the body starts to fail to cope. Blood sugar levels drop and at this stage physiological disorders, such as heart disease, can develop over time.

Symptoms of stress in sport

Psychological symptoms are likely to accompany the physiological symptoms of stress identified above. People under stress often feel worried and unable to make decisions. The worry over feeling stressed can cause even more stress/anxiety. Many people who are experiencing stress feel a sense of losing control and not being able to concentrate.

Sue Challis, the 1984 world champion trampolinist, became very anxious, to the point of crying, when she felt under pressure. Her stress levels seemed to be linked to her confidence level at a particular time – if training was going well, her stress levels were consequently low. She described symptoms such as loss of appetite and sleeplessness during her build-up to a competition. She also tended to become mentally exhausted because of her fear of failing. 'On a good run-up to a competition I suffer from panic a week beforehand, then I'm all right from then on in – it gets better towards the day.'

IN THE NEWS

Former England cricketer Marcus Trescothick suffered anxiety attacks from the age of ten. At the age of 32, Trescothick pulled out of England's 2006–07 Ashes tour with depression that was later diagnosed as stress-related anxiety attacks.

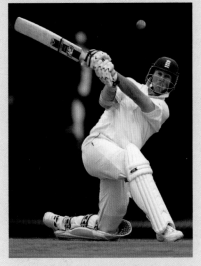

▲ Figure 5.4.3 Sports performers are increasingly being diagnosed with stress-related anxiety attacks

Stress/anxiety management techniques

Two types of state anxiety have been recognised:

- cognitive anxiety (stress response of the mind)
- somatic anxiety (stress response of the body).

The ways in which sports performers can control the amount of stress can be cognitive or somatic or, in many cases, a mixture of both.

Management of cognitive anxiety can affect the somatic anxiety, and vice versa. Controlling the heart rate using relaxation methods can make us feel more positive about performing. Positive thinking can, in turn, control our heart rate. Setting goals can also affect stress/anxiety levels.

Cognitive stress management techniques

Positive thinking/self-talk

Sports performers often use positive thinking not only to motivate themselves or to 'psych themselves up' but also to control stress and self-doubt that often cause stress in sport. Positive thinking is a cognitive process when sports performers think about attaining success and the prospect of winning rather than losing.

Self-talk is about being positive about your past performances and your future strategies by talking to yourself and this can help your confidence and ultimately your performance in sport.

Negative thought stopping

Many sports performers use negative self-talk: 'I will never get any better'; 'I am going to drop this catch'. Instructions aimed at yourself can be directed towards technique or towards your emotions. Halting this negativity is often called 'negative thought stopping'.

RESEARCH IN FOCUS

When sports people become more anxious, they are less able to distinguish between positive and negative thoughts. The negative thoughts become the focus of attention. Negative thoughts, according to sports psychologist Martens (1980), can be placed into five categories:

1 Worry about performance, especially about comparing with others.

2 Inability to make decisions because there is too much going on in your mind.

3 Preoccupation with physical feelings such as fatigue.

4 Thinking about what will happen if you lose and the consequences (such as disapproval).

5 Thoughts of not having enough ability to do well – too much self-criticism.

As performers become more skilful, they tend not to consciously talk to themselves or conscientiously think about the details of their planned actions so much. To ensure that performers consciously know what they are trying to achieve, it is best for them, in training, to use self-talk that is positive and to stop negative thinking. Words or phrases can be used in training to help skill development – in rugby it could be 'fast hands'; in hockey it could be 'steady'.

Rational thinking

This again is a cognitive process often used by successful athletes. How stressed a sports performer feels depends on their response to a given stressor. For example, a performer who fears being physically hurt is stressed about meeting the demands of the situation and limiting the damage. Perception is the key here because it is the interpretation of the situation that dictates the level of stress that the performer experiences.

Rational thinking is about challenging any negative thoughts we may have by looking at the logical and real aspects of a situation. Athletes may be rational by thinking about their extensive training programme and how this will prepare them for any pain or discomfort associated with their sport. The athlete may think rationally by realising that very few athletes are actually physically damaged by any situation and if they are then it is often not a life or death situation. Rational thinking will take into consideration the planning that has taken place before the event or competition and also weigh up the chances of winning in a realistic way.

Mental rehearsal and imagery

Mental rehearsal

Mental rehearsal, sometimes called mental practice, is a strategy adopted by many sportsmen and women. By mentally rehearsing, you form a mental image of the skill or event that you are about to perform. No physical movements are involved in mental rehearsal. Some performers find mental rehearsal easier than others, but the technique can be improved with practice. Mental rehearsal is used either to learn a new skill or to improve existing skills and to control stress/anxiety.

Key term

Mental rehearsal: the technique of forming a mental image of the skill or event that you are about to perform.

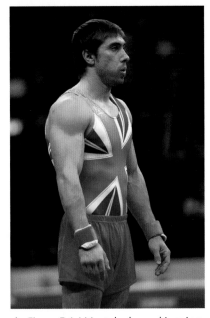

▲ Figure 5.4.4 Mental rehearsal is going through the activity in your mind, which helps control stress levels

For example, before performing the serial skill of a floor routine, a gymnast will go through the routine in his mind by creating a mental image of each stage of the routine – this may make him more confident in his performance. Before taking a penalty kick, a soccer player may visualise her kick and the desired result, which can control stress.

For the novice, mental rehearsal may well improve confidence and help to control arousal levels. Research has shown that if a performer concentrates on successful movements rather than unsuccessful ones, they experience a degree of optimism.

Evaluation

By combining physical and mental practice, all performers, especially those who are already skilled, will be able to improve their performance. To maximise the effects of mental rehearsal, teachers and coaches should encourage the performer to mentally rehearse successful movements away from the heat of competition. Mental rehearsal should include as much fine detail as possible. The performer should also be encouraged to mentally rehearse during rest periods between practice sessions.

RESEARCH IN FOCUS

Many researchers have concluded that mental rehearsal that is combined with physical practice can lead to high performance levels and less stress. Mental practice can help to visualise faults and the correction of those faults can help with controlling arousal levels and can activate the body to respond to particular cues.

Study hint

Consider a range of examples of how imagery might help and how mental rehearsal might help in controlling stress.

Imagery

The technique of imagery can help to improve concentration and develop confidence, and to ensure the correct response. Imagery differs from mental rehearsal because it involves the formation of mental images that are often unrelated to the actual activity. Imagery has a number of uses:

- To create a mental picture to get the feeling of movement or to try to capture an emotional feeling.

- To create pictures of escape – we could imagine ourselves in a much more relaxed place, such as lying on a beach in a far-away country. The creation of mental pictures is called visualisation. Many top sports people use this method to help them control stress/anxiety.

- To recall sounds as well as pictures – to hear the sound of the cricket ball being hit by your bat or the 'swish' of the ball as it goes through the net in basketball.

- To try to feel what it is like to perform a skill – a successful tackle in rugby or the exhilaration of running fast.

- To try to imagine your emotions – to feel the happiness and sense of achievement in saving a penalty or holing a putt in golf.

Activity

Visualisation: close your eyes and visualise yourself performing your sport. Try to imagine performing just one skill, such as hitting a forehand in tennis or kicking a ball in football.

Imagery: to escape, close your eyes and imagine that you are in a comfortable place, such as lying on a deserted beach under the afternoon sun.

Now answer the following questions:

1 How effective is your visualisation and can you easily maintain a mental picture of performance?

2 Did you find imagery easy or difficult to carry out and what emotional responses were you aware of?

There are two forms of imagery:

- external imagery – seeing yourself from outside your body, as if you were in a film
- internal imagery – seeing yourself from within.

Internal imagery is probably more effective than external imagery, but most people prefer to use one method over the other. To be effective in using imagery, the following points should be taken into consideration:

- Relax in a comfortable, warm setting before you attempt to practise imagery.
- If you want to improve a skill by using imagery, practise in a real-life situation.
- Imagery exercises should be short but frequent.
- Set goals for each session – for example, concentrate on imagining the feel of a tennis serve in one short session.
- Construct a programme for your training in imagery.
- Evaluate your programme at regular intervals. Use the sports imagery evaluation described below to help you assess your training.

Activity

Imagery evaluation: imagine a situation, providing as much detail from your imagination as possible to make the image as real as you can. Then rate your imagery on a scale of 1–5 (1 being not much and 5 being very much) according to:

1 how vividly you saw the image
2 how clearly you heard the sounds
3 how vividly you felt the body movements
4 how clearly you felt the mood or emotions of the situation.

The higher your rating, the better you are at using imagery.

Mindfulness

Mindfulness is an old technique that has attracted more attention over the past few years, for managing stress/anxiety. Athletes in many sports are turning to this technique to cope with the high mental demands of their chosen activity.

Key term

Mindfulness: used as a therapeutic technique, often involving meditation, with the individual taking into account the present. It concerns our environmental awareness and our relationships with others at a particular point in time.

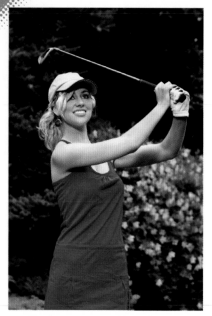

▲ Figure 5.4.5 Mindfulness is about attending and appreciating the present

We are all too busy with everyday life, along with tackling myriad emotions and thoughts, and we often fail to take in how we feel and what we are doing in the present. We reflect on what we have done and what we are going to do, yet we rarely take into full consideration the present and the world around us in a particular moment in time. Mindfulness is about paying attention to the present moment, often involving meditation, and this can be linked to our mental well-being and our ability to control stress/anxiety.

A golfer, for example, may well be worrying about the next hole or be anxious about a previous shot. If this golfer practised mindfulness, then she might try to put these worries aside and concentrate on the peaceful surroundings or the 'flow' of her current golf swing.

Mindfulness can lead to the 'peak flow experience' or zone of optimum functioning explored in Chapter 5.1 of Book 1.

IN THE NEWS

In October 2015, an all-party parliamentary group considered the use of mindfulness and concluded that meditation courses, unrelated to religion, should be made available to 580,000 people who suffered recurrent relapses into depression, at an initial cost of £10 million. This group recommended that the government should train 1,200 new meditation teachers and there should be more mindfulness taught in schools following evidence that it reduces misbehaviour and can improve GCSE results.

Source: 'Mindful nation UK', Report by the Mindfulness All-party Parliamentary Group, October 2015

RESEARCH IN FOCUS

Research by Baer *et al.*, called 'Weekly change in mindfulness and perceived stress in a mindfulness-based stress reduction program' (2012), into individuals with high levels of stress found significant improvement in perceived levels of stress after a course of mindfulness. The findings of this research were consistent with other studies showing that changes in mindfulness 'precede changes in perceived stress'.

Mindfulness and sport performance has recently become a popular topic in sports psychology research. Enhancing the current personal awareness by a sports performer can affect peak sport performance (Jackson and Csikszentmihalyi, 1999; Ravizza, 2002).

Research by Aherne *et al.* (2011) and Kee and Wang (2008) has suggested that mindfulness exercises can help to generate 'flow', or help performers to enhance the focus on a particular sporting task or event.

Cue utilisation

Mindfulness, mental rehearsal and imagery can all lead a sports performer to take note of important signals or cues from the environment that may help them in their performance. This is known as cue utilisation.

Attention is more effective if the performer concentrates on cues that are relevant at the particular time – maintaining focus and not being distracted are features displayed by top performers. If cues in the environment are not used effectively, the sports person fails to gather relevant information from around the field of play – for instance, a hockey player might not be aware of movements off the ball that will affect her next pass. There is also the danger that the player could be distracted too easily by irrelevant cues, such as a person in the crowd shouting at them.

The classic work by the psychologist Easterbrook (Easterbrook, J.A. (1959) The effects of emotion on cue utilization and the organization of behavior. Psychological Review, 66, 183–201) proposed the cue utilisation theory, which states that as the athlete's arousal level increases, their attention narrows. The optimum level of arousal is seen as being moderate, because this is when the athlete ignores irrelevant cues but concentrates on the relevant ones. If the arousal levels are too low, then both irrelevant and relevant cues are attended to; if the arousal levels are too high, the irrelevant and relevant cues are ignored and consequently there is a drop in performance.

Goal setting

The setting of goals is an important strategy which teachers, coaches and performers can adopt to control levels of stress/anxiety in sport. Goal setting is often used to increase a performer's motivation and confidence. Participants in sport are often faced with complex and threatening situations and may feel anxious. Goal setting can help to alleviate this anxiety and ultimately enhance performance.

RESEARCH IN FOCUS

According to prominent academics Lock and Latham (1985) in their work with business management, goal setting can affect performance – in sports as well as in management – in four ways:

1 By directing attention.
2 By regulating the amount of effort that is put into a given task.
3 By ensuring effort is sustained until the goal is reached.
4 By motivating people to develop a variety of strategies to reach their goals.

Goal setting is an effective cognitive strategy to manage stress in sport. Many top sports performers recognise their limitations but strive for more success. Therefore, goals set should follow the SMART principle (see Book 1, page 214 for more information on SMART goal setting).

Evaluation

To help a sports person deal with stress/anxiety over the outcome, success may have to be redefined. Personal performance goals may be less stress-inducing than outcome goals and will put the participant in a position of control. Emphasis could shift towards more process-type goals – for example, to develop sports performance skills or strategies. A move away from outcome goals – for example, whether you will win a particular sports competition – may make losing bearable and less stressful, thus reducing stress/anxiety. Setting goals such as personal bests can help the sports person to focus on performance and process-type goals.

Activity

Write down some possible long-term goals related to your sport, your coaching or even your studies. Now try to identify some short-term goals or objectives that might help you achieve your long-term goals. Use all the guidance that was set out in this last section. Are the goals you have set measurable, achievable, specific? Are they outcome goals, performance goals or process-oriented goals?

Evaluation

Goals need to be measurable. Their measurement will give information about success, in itself a motivating factor, and will give useful information about setting further goals. There is nothing worse for a performer than not knowing how they are progressing, so accurate feedback is essential.

Goal setting can also alleviate stress in sport at lower levels of performance. For example, someone who might wish to become fitter and healthier may set short-term goals leading to longer term goals. Setting goals such as being able to walk a couple of miles first before being able to jog the same distance may limit the stress experienced because the short-term goal is achievable for most people.

Different types of goals

Different types of goals will affect the performer in different ways.

- Outcome goals are related to the end result. Sports people and their instructors often set goals to win or are concerned with the outcome of the competition.
- Performance goals are concerned with performance judged against other performances – perhaps a certain time to be achieved in order to better the last time recorded. These goals are related to specific behaviours. Performance goals may affect outcome goals.
- Process-oriented goals concentrate on the performer's technique and tactics – in other words, what a performer has to do to be more successful.

Extend your knowledge

Goal difficulty

Research has shown that setting difficult goals leads to better performance than setting medium or easy goals. There is evidence to suggest that goals that are set just beyond reach produce a better performance than those that are achieved with ease. If the task to be achieved is complex, with many perceptual requirements, goal setting becomes less effective in the short term, but the strategies that have been tried and failed could be useful in the long term. Generally speaking, goals must be achievable but challenging. If goals are set too easy, motivation will soon decline.

Goal specificity

Clearly defined goals usually lead to better performance. Simply saying 'do your best' is not good enough – targets need to be better defined. Evaluation of goals is also difficult if the goals have not been clearly defined. Sports involving objective measurements, such as time, are easier to make specific, but it is possible to set specific goals in most activities.

Other factors affecting goal setting

Long-term and short-term goals

Achievement of long-term goals is a progressive process and must start with achieving short-term goals. Many athletes use realistic target dates to help them achieve their short-term goals. Short-term goals provide a greater opportunity for success, which can reinforce positive feelings and in turn help to control stress/anxiety levels.

Sharing decision-making

Goals that are set through negotiation and agreement are far more effective than externally set goals. The participant will have a sense of ownership over the goal setting and will be better motivated to achieve. Goal setting is also likely to be fairer and more realistic if all parties involved have an input.

Somatic stress management techniques

Somatic stress management techniques involve relaxation exercises that concern the body's muscles rather than concentrating on the mind.

Relaxation

Relaxation mainly controls somatic anxiety but can also work on cognitive anxiety. It is useful to go through some relaxation exercises before attempting to train yourself in mental exercises such as imagery. Relaxation can help players adopt a calm and positive attitude before a game. Relaxation requires practice, just as mental imagery does, and practices are best if they are progressive.

Self-directed relaxation needs plenty of practice to be effective. The athlete, with help from the coach, concentrates on each muscle group separately and relaxes it. Eventually the athlete can perform this without help, or perhaps with the aid of a pre-recorded tape. The aim of self-relaxation is to take as little time as possible to become fully relaxed so that eventually it will take just a few moments. This time factor is crucial if the athlete is to be able to use the strategy just before or during competition. This technique is effective if the athlete can be aware of the muscles to be relaxed – some have more self-awareness than others, although this can be improved over time.

Progressive muscular relaxation

This technique was developed by Jacobsen in 1932 and is sometimes referred to as the Jacobsen technique. It is a much lengthier process initially than self-relaxation, but can be very effective. The technique is concerned with learning to be aware of and to 'feel' the tension in the muscles and then to get rid of this tension by 'letting go'.

Progressive muscular relaxation becomes more effective with practice. Although this technique may take longer to master, many top sports people have found it most helpful, especially leading up to competition. It has also helped many to achieve a better night's sleep before competition and can be good preparation for imagery exercises.

Biofeedback

Biofeedback gives an anxious person in sport the opportunity to understand their physiological responses to stress. When an athlete becomes stressed or anxious, some of the changes can be as follows:

- an increase in heart rate
- rapid breathing
- increase or decrease in skin temperature
- an increase in muscle tension.

Biofeedback is a process by which different kinds of equipment are used to collect information on a number of physiological responses. Biofeedback information or data include heart rate, blood pressure and respiration rates. The performer records this information, possibly reacting to it in different ways. They are aware of how their body is working at a given time and this affects the emotions and levels of stress they experience.

Sports coaches often use this method to encourage an athlete to deal effectively, and with less stress/anxiety, to the body's reaction to exercise. For example, a heart monitor may be used to collect data on heart rate during exercise or at rest. If the athlete realises that their heart rate is

Activity

Sit on the floor with your legs straight out in front of you. Tense the muscles of your right leg by a dorsiflex action of your ankle joint (pull your toes up towards your knee using your leg and foot muscles). Develop as much tension as possible and hold it for about five seconds, concentrating on what it feels like. Then completely relax your leg muscles and let your foot go floppy, concentrating on what the relaxed muscles feel like. Now try to relax your muscles even further. How does your leg feel? It should feel much more relaxed.

increased too much at the beginning of the race and is causing too much stress/anxiety, they can develop strategies to combat this stress response by using slower, deeper breathing techniques and mental imagery, for example.

Biofeedback can help with imagery or visualisation to reduce stress and to enhance relaxation. For example, if blood pressure is raised too much in a situation where there is an audience and this causes stress/anxiety, the athlete can maintain focus by directing their attention to a specific aspect of their performance and this can help them in developing mental cues to eliminate distractions, such as the noise of the crowd.

In some sports, biofeedback can involve simulation machines to help the sports performer prepare for the event both physically and emotionally, often controlling the level of stress/anxiety they experience and therefore managing stress effectively. For example, in the winter sport of bobsleigh, athletes have used a computer-controlled simulator to precisely replicate or copy the sensations that may be experienced on a specific bobsleigh track. The biofeedback data, such as heart rate during a run with the athlete experiencing the effect of the gravitational forces, are noted. When the athlete knows that a particularly difficult corner of the course lies ahead, they may experience high stress/anxiety. Once the athlete realises this, they can employ strategies to control this stress/anxiety, turning it into a positive rather than a negative aspect by anticipating when it will occur in the 'real' world, and therefore they will be more prepared for the actual event.

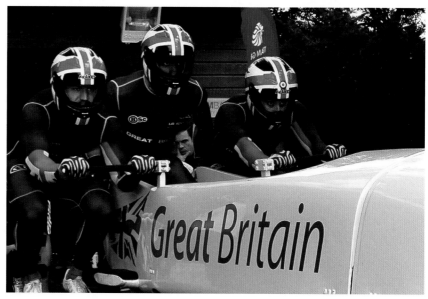

▲ Figure 5.4.6 Biofeedback can help prepare athletes for anticipated anxiety-inducing events

Biofeedback teaches the individual how to control the brain's activity and maintain the proper brainwave levels to achieve a calm and focused state. By returning the body to a healthier physiological state, the feelings of doubt and confusion, as well as the feelings of fear and panic throughout the body, are removed.

Centring technique

Centring or centering is a technique combining both somatic and cognitive responses that is used by sports performers to control stress/anxiety. This technique is similar to mindfulness in that you focus on the here and now, and concentration is shifted to the centre of the body (just behind the navel). The mind recognises that the body is responding to a stressful event in a particular way – for example, by increasing heart rate or sweating and shaking. This feedback occurs as a result of energy flowing throughout the body. The athlete, through the centring technique, will then redirect this energy to the centre of their body and thus achieve a calm and steady state.

The basic skill to master for effective centring practice is to focus on breathing. You pay particular attention to each inhalation and exhalation and you take note of every sensation that occurs as the air flows in and out of the nostrils, and as the air enters the lungs. With each breath you may notice the sensations of heat, cold and the speed of the air flow.

To begin this practice, simply start in a quiet place with no distractions and focus your attention on the rate of breathing while maintaining a slow, steady pace. In order for this to become a useful skill on the sports field, you should practise this technique regularly so that you can use it automatically, thus reducing stress/anxiety and distraction when you need to most, during sports competition or training.

Activity

Centring:

1   Stand, sit or lie down and try to feel physically relaxed.
2   Close your eyes and breathe steadily. Try to let go of any inner tension, especially in the upper part of your body.
3   Breathe in deeply through your nose and from your abdomen/stomach. Be aware of any upper body tension.
4   Breathe out through your mouth and let the tension disappear. Focus on the feeling of heaviness in your abdomen/stomach area.
5   Keep breathing in and out steadily and deeply. Now focus all your attention to the centre of your body – just behind your navel.
6   Keep concentrating on the centre point and try to feel calm, controlled and relaxed.
7   Imagine all of the energy in your body flowing into your centre point.
8   When you begin to feel stressed in sport, turn your attention to your centre to remind yourself that you have balance and control. Then breathe in and out deeply at least five times. Continue to concentrate on your centre and feel the sensation of being in control and calm.

Breathing control

The most basic way to lower stress/anxiety and to try to relax is using a somatic technique of controlled breathing, mainly through deep, slow breaths.

Deep breathing has many important benefits. It ensures that you get enough oxygen so your body can exercise effectively. By getting more oxygen into your body, you will be more relaxed and feel more in control and less stressed. This will give you greater confidence and enable you to combat any negative thoughts. Focusing on your breathing can also help to take your mind off things that are making you anxious.

For athletes who participate in sports that involve a series of short performances, such as tennis and golf, deep breathing can help and should be a part of the routines between short performances – for example, in golf walking between shots, or between serves in tennis.

Activity

1   Breathe in through your nose, out through your mouth.
2   Breathe from your stomach, not from your shoulders.
3   Focus on relaxing thoughts as you breathe or on words such as calm, smooth, control, relax, etc.

155

Summary

- Stress often arises as a result of an athlete's perception that their capabilities may not match the demands imposed upon them. Stressors include competition, conflict, frustration, climate, injury and evaluation in sport.
- The ways in which sports performers can control the amount of stress can be cognitive or somatic or, in many cases, a mixture of both.
- Positive thinking is a cognitive process when sports performers think about attaining success and the prospect of winning rather than losing. Rational thinking is about challenging any negative thoughts we may have by looking at the logical and real aspects of a situation. Mental rehearsal can help to visualise faults and the correction of those faults can help with controlling arousal levels and can activate the body to respond to particular cues. The technique of imagery can help to improve concentration and develop confidence. Mindfulness is about paying attention to the present moment and this can be linked to our mental well-being and our ability to control stress/anxiety. SMART goal setting is often used to motivate, boost confidence and help with stress/anxiety control.
- Somatic stress management techniques involve relaxation exercises that concern the body muscles rather than concentrating on the mind. Progressive muscular relaxation is concerned with learning to be aware of and to 'feel' the tension in the muscles and then to get rid of this tension by 'letting go'. Biofeedback is a process by which different kinds of equipment are used to collect information on a number of physiological responses. Centring is similar to mindfulness in that you focus on the here and now and concentration is shifted to the centre of the body (just behind the navel).

Check your understanding

1 What is meant by the term stress in sport?
2 What are the main causes of stress in sport?
3 What is meant by cognitive stress management techniques?
4 What is meant by somatic stress management techniques?
5 What examples can you give of these different techniques?

Practice questions

1 Sports performers often experience stress when competing. Using examples, explain the causes of stress during sports competition. (8 marks)
2 Explain how three different cognitive stress management techniques could be used by a sports performer during competition. (6 marks)
3 Discuss the use of mindfulness in controlling stress in sport. (4 marks)
4 Explain how somatic stress management techniques can help athletes control levels of stress/anxiety in sport. (8 marks)
5 Explain the somatic stress management technique of biofeedback in sport. (5 marks)

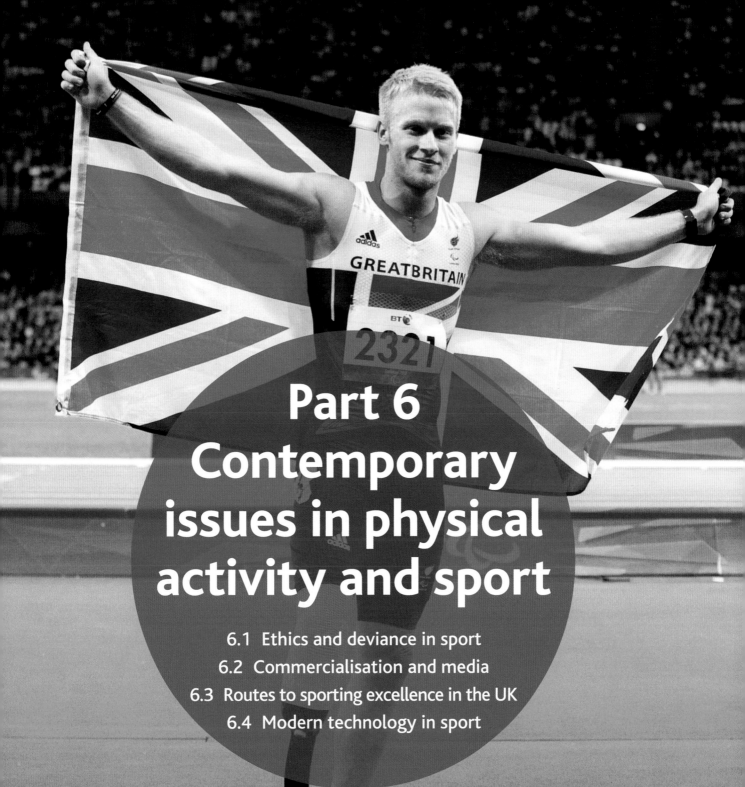

Part 6
Contemporary issues in physical activity and sport

6.1 Ethics and deviance in sport
6.2 Commercialisation and media
6.3 Routes to sporting excellence in the UK
6.4 Modern technology in sport

6.1 Ethics and deviance in sport

Understanding the specification

By the end of this chapter you should:

- have an understanding of drugs and doping in sport and legal supplements versus illegal drugs and doping
- recognise the reasons why elite performers use illegal drugs/doping and the consequences/implications to society, sport and performers
- know the strategies to stop the use of illegal drugs and doping
- have developed your understanding of the implications to society, sport and performers, and know the strategies to prevent violence, both for players and for spectators
- be aware about gambling in sport and about match fixing, bribery and illegal sports betting.

Key terms

Ethics: rules that dictate an individual's conduct. They form a system of rules that groups and societies are judged on. An ethic in sport would be that athletes stick to the spirit of the rules of the game.

Deviance: a word that describes unacceptable behaviour within a culture. Any behaviour that differs from the perceived social or legal norm is seen as deviant.

We like to see sport associated with fair play, but due to its competitive nature and the pressures on performers, coaches and administrators, sports activities can be affected by poor **ethics** and behaviour. This chapter will explore the unethical factors of illegal performance-enhancing drug taking and the implications of this, together with the strategies to control and combat the use of these illegal substances.

Deviance in sport, which is often a result of the drive to win – occasionally at 'all costs', can also be viewed as unethical. Violent behaviour shown by some participants and spectators is a feature of modern competitive sport and we will investigate the strategies that might prevent such behaviour. Gambling in sport, although historically prevalent, is now more sophisticated and a main attraction for those who follow major sports in the UK. Gambling can bring with it illegal practices, such as match fixing, to try to make 'a fast buck' and sadly there have been incidents in major sports of bribery and corruption.

Drugs and doping in sport

Both illegal consumption of performance-enhancing drugs and **blood doping** have been a feature in many sports and are examples of deviance. The drug-taking revelations surrounding the Russian athletics team in 2015, along with high-profile sports performers such as the US cyclist Lance Armstrong, make this a contemporary topic for exploration. The use of drugs, whether recreational (for example, cannabis) or performance-enhancing (for example, anabolic steroids) can seriously affect your health and well-being.

Blood doping

Blood doping is a process that increases a person's red blood cell count. A greater number of red blood cells means that higher volumes of haemoglobin are present. Blood doping therefore allows extra oxygen to be transported to the working muscles, resulting in a higher level of performance, without the use of the anaerobic energy systems. It commonly involves the removal of approximately two pints of the athlete's blood several weeks prior to competition. The blood is then frozen until 1–2 days before the competition, when it is thawed and injected back into the athlete.

Blood doping is most commonly used by endurance athletes, such as distance runners and cyclists. Studies have shown that blood doping can improve the performance of endurance athletes.

Extend your knowledge

The possible side effects of blood doping are:

- increased blood viscosity
- increased risk of heart attack
- pulmonary embolism (a blockage, which can be fat, air or a blood clot, of the pulmonary artery)
- cerebral embolism (a blockage, formed elsewhere in the body, which becomes lodged in an artery within or leading to the brain)
- cerebrovascular accident (stroke)
- infections and risk of blood-borne diseases (Hepatitis C, B and HIV)
- allergic reaction.

More information can be found in Book 1, Chapter 2.1.

Examples of performance-enhancing drugs

Drugs are often used to enhance performance illegally in sport and have been widely reported recently in many sports. We need to develop an understanding of the main performance-enhancing drugs:

- Anabolic steroids: these enable sports people to train harder and longer and often lead to increasing their strength and aggression.
- Beta blockers: these help to control the heart rate and keep the athlete calm.
- Stimulants: these work as a brain stimulant, which increases alertness for sports people. An example is amphetamines.

Other prohibited classes of substances are:

- narcotic analgesics
- anabolic agents
- diuretics
- peptide hormones, mimetics and analogues
- substances with anti-oestrogenic activity
- masking agents.

Prohibited methods are:

- enhancement of oxygen transfer
- blood doping
- the administration of products that enhance the uptake, transport and delivery of oxygen
- pharmacological, chemical and physical manipulation
- gene doping.

Classes of prohibited substances in certain circumstances include:

- alcohol
- cannabinoids
- local anaesthetics
- glucocorticosteroids.

See Book 1, Chapter 2.1 for a recap on prohibited substances.

Legal supplements versus illegal drugs and doping in sport

Many sports performers use legal supplements to maximise training and performance in sport. Even these could be viewed by some people as cheating since they aid performance, but they are accepted by sports administrators because they do not significantly enhance performance or significantly affect the performer's health and well-being.

Legal supplements – for example, vitamins and minerals – are now freely available, many over the internet. However, some manufacturers' claims that they help sports performance are based on questionable or conflicting research. Such supplements may not be safe to use, particularly in high doses. Little is known about the long-term effects of some dietary substances and prolonged use could be causing damage to health.

The philosophy of sport is for fair play and the taking of legal supplements is still within the bounds of acceptable fair play, whereas taking illegal substances is not deemed to be so.

Extend your knowledge

Legal supplements include bicarbonate, beta-hydroxy-beta-methylbutyrate (HMB), creatine, calcium, carbohydrate powders and gels, glucosamine and chondroitin, intramuscular iron, intramuscular vitamin B12, liquid meal replacements, melatonin, recovery formulas, sports energy bars, skimmed milk powder, sports drinks, specific vitamins and minerals.

See Book 1, Chapter 2.1 for more detail on legal supplements versus illegal drugs and doping in sport.

Advantages of taking legal supplements

Dietary supplements are used in addition to a normal diet to improve general health and well-being or to enhance sporting performance. Supplements can include sports drinks or vitamins, which claim to help with building muscle, increasing stamina, weight control, improving flexibility, rehydrating or aiding recovery after exercise. Dietary supplements can be found in tablet, powder or liquid form.

Evaluation

Illegal drugs and blood doping can result in dramatic improvement in performance or shorten recovery in training and between competitions. However, by taking these substances the performer is breaking the law and potentially putting their health at severe risk.

Legal substances do not put an individual's or a sport's reputation at risk; if others find out that you are taking legal supplements, you are unlikely to be judged harshly. There are no punishments for taking legal supplements, whereas the punishments for being caught taking performance-enhancing drugs or for blood doping are increasingly severe.

Supplements are used by sports performers, athletes and bodybuilders to help increase strength, performance and recovery. They are available in numerous different forms, ranging from multivitamins and minerals through to protein, creatine and various other **ergogenic aids**, which are intended to enhance performance. More detail on ergogenic aids can be found in Book 1, Chapter 2.1.

Before individuals opt to take any form of supplement they should ensure their diet is healthy, balanced and suits their sport. Some people take supplementary creatine, which is a high-energy compound that helps to store and provide energy. It is hugely popular with sports performers. It is intended to help you train for longer and also to increase performance during high-intensity exercise.

Staying well hydrated during exercise and training is extremely important as dehydration is detrimental to sports performance. Simply drinking water is a good way of keeping hydrated during exercise periods, although some individuals also opt for energy drinks, particularly those who undertake endurance events such as long-distance running. Many energy drinks contain electrolytes such as sodium, which help to stimulate thirst and encourage drinking, as well as enhancing the body's ability to hold water. In addition, the carbohydrates contained in many energy drinks can give individuals extra energy, which they may need in the latter stages of training, and could also provide extra protein to help prevent muscle loss.

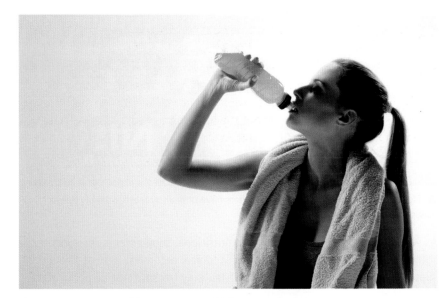

▲ Figure 6.1.1 Many athletes use sports drinks as supplements

The disadvantages of taking legal supplements

Some supplements can present risks to sports performers – they can contain banned substances or can be contaminated during the manufacturing process. Some supplements may not be what they seem and may not contain what is stated on the packet or in the accompanying sales literature.

Sports scientists have raised concerns over the long-term health implications of taking creatine for prolonged periods, as some research has suggested it may have undesirable effects on the digestive system and could also result in muscular and cardiovascular issues as well as potentially increasing the risk of cancer. Many energy drinks are extremely high in sugar and prolonged use can contribute to health issues such as obesity and tooth decay.

IN THE NEWS

In newspaper reports in November 2015, it was reported that some professional footballers had unhealthy teeth and gums, possibly linked to sugary sports drinks. For example, *The Guardian* reported that, despite their bodies being young and fit and their diets being strictly controlled by nutrition experts, professional footballers' teeth were likely to be in worse shape than the average person. As part of a study in the *British Journal of Sports Medicine*, on examination of 187 senior players at eight clubs, dentists found that 37 per cent had 'active dental caries' (cavities), 77 per cent had at least one filling (with, on average, five) and 77 per cent had gingivitis covering at least half their mouths.

You can read the full article from *The Guardian* on 3 November 2015, at www.theguardian.com/football/shortcuts/2015/nov/03/foul-mouthed-why-are-footballers-teeth-so-bad

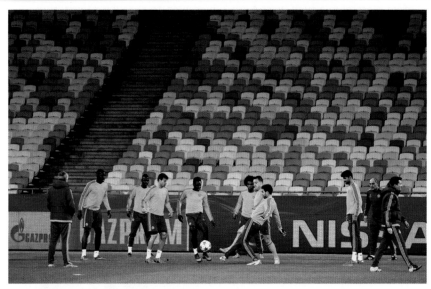

▲ Figure 6.1.2 Many professional footballers have unhealthy teeth, possibly linked to sugary sports drinks

As well as the health issues of taking nutritional supplements for sport, some would argue that there is a philosophical argument against taking supplements – it is not in the spirit of fair play because not all performers have access to such supplements, or the cost may be beyond their reach. Others argue that some supplements are bordering on the illegal and may well contain traces of illegal or banned substances. The purist might argue that simple physical training for your sport, including fitness and skills training, with a normal balanced diet would make a level 'playing field' for sports competition. Many nutritionists agree that a well-planned, balanced diet and regular intake of water are all that is required for a sports performer at most levels of competition. More detail of diet and sport can be found in Book 1, Chapter 2.1.

Study hint

When considering the use of legal supplements versus illegal drugs and doping, make sure that you revise arguments for and against their use in sport and use practical examples to illustrate your answer where appropriate.

Reasons why elite performers use illegal drugs and doping

There is growing evidence that more and more elite performers, especially in athletics, have used illegal drugs or doping.

IN THE NEWS

PERFORMANCE-ENHANCING DRUGS IN ATHLETICS – A SCANDAL

Much of the media have highlighted the alleged misuse of drugs by athletes, especially the Russian athletics team. Leading figures responded to a World Anti-Doping Agency (WADA) commission report in November 2015 which recommended that Russia should be banned from competition. The report examined claims of doping and extortion in Russian athletics and also stated that the Olympics in London in 2012 were 'sabotaged' by Russian athletes taking part despite them being under suspicion. The British Minister for Sport and the Olympics, Tracey Crouch, called the findings an 'extraordinarily dark day for athletics'.

You can read more on this at: www.bbc.co.uk/sport/athletics/34766733

Elite performers are under a tremendous amount of pressure to succeed – from coaches, friends, family, other performers and, of course, themselves. This pressure can affect the performer's judgements and decision-making, resulting in decisions that they will ultimately come to regret. The pressure can lead performers to resort to illegal means to make just enough difference to win. The influence of coaches is often underestimated because they, too, are under pressure to succeed and some strive to bask in the glory of the performers they coach.

Political pressures are another factor in motivating elite performers to take performance-enhancing drugs. Politicians often want to enjoy their nation's success in sport and this can lead to a great deal of pressure on individual athletes and teams to use whatever means at their disposal to win and attain status for their nation. The Russian athletics scandal highlights the pressure put on coaches and athletes recently, but this is not just a contemporary issue. Throughout history, and particularly during the Cold War, nations have put undue, illegal and immoral pressure on sportsmen and women. In the 1970s and 1980s, drug taking was rife among East German sports competitors. This state-sponsored doping regime played a decisive role in the massive success of East German athletes in international competitions, especially in the 1976 Montreal Olympics and the 1980 Moscow Games.

The monetary rewards today are so substantial for winning high-profile sports competition, along with the associated status and future earning capacity. This significant level of reward can motivate sports performers to cheat and to take performance-enhancing drugs. Successful athletes not only receive large amounts of prize money, they also attract lucrative sponsorship deals with global commercial companies.

IN THE NEWS

MO FARAH'S COACH SUSPECTED AS DRUGS CHEAT

In June 2015, BBC's *Panorama* alleged a widespread culture of drug abuse in Alberto Salazar's training camp in Portland, Oregon, USA. Mo Farah had trained at the camp from 2011. The allegations included pills hidden in paperback novels and the doping of a schoolboy prodigy. Mo Farah insisted that he had not taken any banned substances and that Salazar had never suggested he take a banned substance.

You can read more on this story at: www.dailymail.co.uk/sport/sportsnews/article-3109642/Mo-Farah-s-training-partner-Galen-Rupp-coach-Alberto-Salazar-accused-doping.html

Another reason that elite performers take illegal drugs or use blood doping is because some of them think, 'Everyone else is taking them so why shouldn't I?' In some activities, such as competitive cycling, illegal use of sports-enhancing methods has become much more the norm, with a record number of cyclists being caught cheating. Some people in sport promote the idea that because there is so much drug taking and because it is now so hard to detect new and developing substances, you might as well accept drug taking as part of sport. This latter depressing view may not be prevalent, but it shows how difficult it is for those who want sport to be fair and healthy for all to keep sport drug-free.

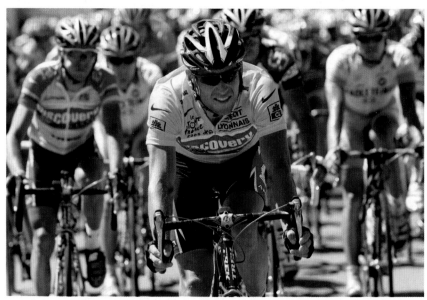

▲ Figure 6.1.3 Rewards and status associated with success can motivate athletes to cheat

Consequences and implications of drugs and doping in sport

When athletes use performance-enhancing drugs, there are consequences and implications for sport, performers and society. In sport, the concept of fair play is severely challenged by this type of cheating. Sportsmen and women who are beaten in competition are increasingly wondering whether they have been beaten fairly, and those who do perform well and gain a world record, for example, may feel that others are looking at their success with suspicion – is this high performance due to hard work, training and talent or down to the influence of illegal drug taking?

We have already explored some of the health issues that are associated with taking drugs and blood doping, so the consequences for athletes may well be severe dangers to health and well-being, and even death. In 2012, for example, the coroner at the time ruled that a fit and healthy woman who collapsed near the finish of the London marathon probably died as a result of taking a legally available performance-enhancing drug.

Sports that have been associated with using illegal methods to improve performance, such as cycling and weightlifting, have been tainted, resulting in a struggle to gain sponsorship and loss of some public support. Sponsors are reluctant to lend their brands to athletes who are under suspicion, while damaging press reports – for example, in athletics – have led to many supporters becoming disaffected with their sport. Each sport is under increasing pressure to 'clean up their act' and to put in place more thorough education programmes combating the use of drugs, and those who test for such illegal substances are having to explore new scientific methods to detect their use.

Since sport can be viewed as a reflection of the culture in which it is played, taking drugs in sport has consequences for the wider society. The traditional view of sport has been that it should involve fair competition and that it is character-building, with athletes striving to do their best but maintaining a sense of decency. The use of illegal drugs and blood doping flies in the face of such a view. Now our society can be seen as corrupt and full of unethical citizens who merely want to succeed 'at all costs', with some political leaders and sports role models reinforcing this view through their illegal and corrupt actions. Society can either respond by continuing to be corrupt and condone drug taking as inevitable, or challenge such behaviours as being unethical and against cultural values. Cynicism can lead to passivity over unethical behaviour in both sport and society – for example, merely accepting that bankers, lawyers and politicians all cheat anyway and 'there is nothing we can do about it'. Nevertheless, some people may view recent allegations of widespread cheating in sport as a 'wake-up call' for society and strive for cleaner and more ethical behaviour in sport and in other aspects of life.

Strategies to stop the use of illegal drugs and doping in sport

WADA is an independent body formed by the International Olympic Committee in 1999 with responsibility for drug testing. WADA draws up the list of banned substances. It also provides assistance to countries' own anti-doping programmes and funds research.

It is likely that manufacturers of illegal performance-enhancing drugs will continue to try to be ahead of the regulators. It is also likely that there are 'undetectable' drugs already in use and that others will be manufactured in the future. There are arguments for the legalisation of drugs in sports because of the problems with detection. Drug testing is a regular part of

Study hint

Be prepared to argue the possible consequences to performers, sport and society of taking illegal drugs and using blood doping in sport.

Activity

Set up a debate in class about the advantages and disadvantages of taking drugs in sport. Summarise the arguments and highlight the consequences of such behaviour to sport, performers and society.

both professional and amateur sports. An athlete can be called for drug testing at any time, in or out of competition. During competition, some sports carry out drug testing on the winning team or top three competitors only; others will test by random selection from all competitors.

IN THE NEWS

DRUG TESTING IN TENNIS

In November 2015, on the eve of the ATP World Tour Finals in London, the *Daily Express* reported how Andy Murray and Roger Federer were calling for more drugs testing and financial investment in the testing process. Andy Murray spoke of the need for more transparency and more money to be invested in the anti-doping process given the prize money that can be won by professional tennis players today. More money, he claimed, would improve the ability to catch anyone cheating and increase the trust of the public.

You can read the full article from the *Daily Express* on 13 November 2015, at: www.express.co.uk/sport/tennis/619299/Andy-Murray-Roger-Federer-drug-testing-tennis-news-gossip

Extend your knowledge

Drug testing via a urine sample

When called for a drugs test, the athlete provides a urine sample (in view of an official of the same gender), which they then split into two bottles and seal. A code number is attached to the bottle and recorded. After the sample, the athlete must complete a medical declaration which records all medicines they have taken over the last week. It is important that the athlete records everything, from over-the-counter medicines to supplements and prescribed drugs. If any of these substances are on the prohibited list, the athlete must hold a Therapeutic Use Exemption (TUE). The competitor, representative and official all check the form before the official and athlete sign it and both parties are given a copy. The samples are then sent to a registered laboratory (if there is not one on site), where sample A is tested using gas chromatography (which uses separation techniques to divide the contents of the sample) and mass spectrometry (which provides the exact molecular specification of the compounds). If a positive result is found with sample A, the athlete is notified before sample B is also tested. The athlete or their representative is entitled to be present at the unsealing and testing of the second sample. If this, too, is positive, the relevant sporting organisations are notified and it is their responsibility to decide what penalties or bans are to be imposed.

As well as drug testing it is important that athletes and their coaches are educated about drugs and blood doping so that they fully understand the implications in terms of both health and the rule of law. Governing bodies of sport all have education programmes and information about performance-enhancing drugs, their consequences and how to avoid them.

The widespread use of performance-enhancing drugs has resulted in outrage from 'clean' athletes, coaches and administrators. One way of trying to prevent the illegal misuse of drugs is to create and reinforce a culture of keeping sport free from drugs cheats. This can then put pressure on athletes if their peers, coaches and all who support and organise sport speak up against the taking of performance-enhancing drugs. If the performers', coaches' and organisers' reputations are at risk, it is more unlikely that they will become involved in illegal practices.

Another strategy that works well in combating drug use is for punishments to be much more rigorous and longer lasting. In 2015 WADA doubled the ban for athletes found guilty of doping to four years, with athletes banned for life if they test positive again. Stronger powers are sought by administrators within the sport to punish coaches and those who encourage the taking of drugs or doping to enhance sports performance. These stricter punishments may lead to fewer incidents of drug misuse, but alone they are unlikely to stamp out the practice altogether. Athletes who know that if they are caught they will be stripped of their achievements, such as gold medals in the Olympics, may then think twice before taking performance-enhancing drugs or resorting to blood doping. The threat of a whole nation being banned from an international major competition might result in fewer countries condoning and supporting drug taking in sport.

Violence in sport

Violence in sport is an issue that, along with drug cheats, often graces the back and front pages of our national newspapers. In this section, we will explore the causes for this example of deviance in sport in relation to players and spectators, the implications of violence and strategies to prevent it.

> **Key term**
>
> **Violence:** intense physical force that is directed towards harming another individual or groups of individuals and can cause injury or death.

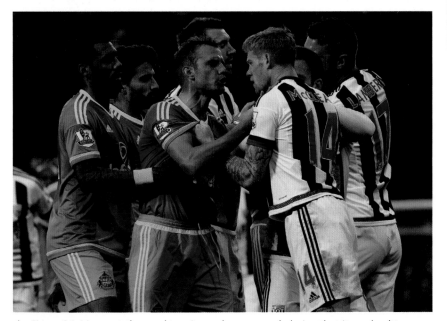

▲ Figure 6.1.4 In sport the need to win can be so overwhelming that it can lead to aggressive or violent conduct

Causes of violence in sport

Sport is often a very competitive activity and the 'win at all costs' mentality is prevalent. The desire to win can be so overwhelming that it can lead to aggressive or violent conduct. Sports teams and individuals are recognised as representatives – for example, of a town or a country – and those who also associate themselves with that town or country can be fiercely protective, which can result in violence among spectators as well as with the performers themselves.

Psychologically, we have investigated aggression in sport in Book 1, Chapter 5.1. We have found that performers will be aggressive if they feel threatened or are frustrated by events. Some sports attract more violence than others because of the nature of the sport itself – for example, the very physical sports such as American football, rugby or ice hockey. High levels of competition can cause individuals to experience significant arousal (see Book 1, Chapter 5.1 for more detail), which heightens emotional responses that can lead to violence.

Violence in sport cannot be isolated from society and its norms and values. Violent crime and behaviour are features of our society, and sport often reflects this by the way it is played and the way supporters behave in the sports environment. The consumption of alcohol or social drugs can also affect supporters' behaviour, while for sports performers the taking of performance-enhancing steroids, such as anabolic steroids, can cause heightened aggression or 'roid rage'.

Rivalries between different groups can lead to violence between individuals who see themselves as 'agents' for their group and who feel a need to protect their group and to assume dominance over other groups. Supporters from a particular football team, for example, might become violent against opposing supporters because of the competition's perceived importance in representing their town, country or simply the group to which they belong. Supporters seeing violence on the field of play might copy that violence because we are more likely to copy the behaviour of role models or significant others – see Chapter 5.1 on aggression in sport in Book 1.

Violence can be due to many factors, both as a participant and as a spectator. Rivalries, between individuals, teams, communities and religions, make up one group of factors. The media can increase tensions by reporting negative aspects of behaviour or simply by reinforcing the rivalries that already exist. The increasing influence of social media can cause disputes to escalate and has even resulted in organised rival supporter fights before football matches. The perception of unfairness or poor officiating can cause frustration for players and spectators and this can lead to violence as a way of releasing this frustration (see frustration-aggression hypothesis in Book 1, Chapter 5.1). The behaviour of individuals in group or team situations can change because they may perceive that they have ceased to be accountable or responsible individuals and now lack individual identity – in other words, they have 'become the group' rather than being an individual. In psychology this is called **deindividuation**.

Key term

Deindividuation: when you lose your sense of being an individual; this can cause violent behaviour.

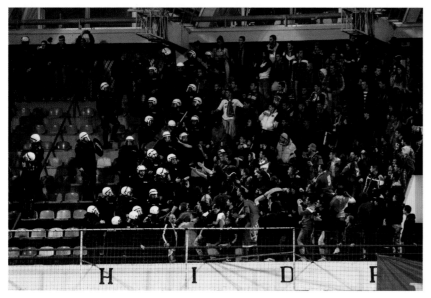

▲ Figure 6.1.5 Supporters may be violent due to deindividuation

If your behaviour is defined by the group to which you belong, you might feel that you cannot be held responsible. For example, you might get into a fight with rival fans at a boxing match because you feel you should show loyalty to your group and believe that you cannot be held responsible or be punished as an individual. Some coaches build on this deindividuation by accentuating the players' team obligations rather than individual responsibilities to encourage violent behaviour that might unsettle opponents, and win possession in a team game, for example.

RESEARCH IN FOCUS

In June 2000 Peter Marsh of the Social Issues Research Centre in Oxford explored sport and group hostilities.

In countries where there are sectarian or cultural group divisions, these are often the basis for clashes between fans. In Italy, regional divisions are the source of rivalries, and in Spain, echoes of the civil war reverberate around matches between Real Madrid and Athletic Bilbao, with Bilbao drawing support among militant anti-Fascists across the country.

You can read more on this subject at http://news.bbc.co.uk/1/hi/world/europe/797601.stm

Implications of violence in sport

Many people believe that sport should be recognised as a mirror to our society and behaviour within sport is influenced by society's norms and values via socialisation (see Book 1, Chapter 5.1 on attitudes and socialisation). Therefore, if violence is to be tackled in sport, then violent behaviour in society should be tackled.

Another implication for society is that watching sport are spectators who relish the idea of violence in the spectacle before them and that part of the entertainment is the violence in some activities, such as boxing and rugby. The laws society sets to control violence and to protect individual citizens might then be applied to all sports situations. Thus, a violent action on the field of play should be treated the same as a violent act out on the streets and the law should be applied equally vigorously.

People who follow sport and directly spectate at sports events are more inclined to violence in certain situations. For example, during the football World Cup in 2010 there was a surge in domestic violence, mainly against women, although there were also incidents of violence against men by women (see 'Research in Focus' below). This domestic violence cannot be linked to the sport itself, in this case football; the causes are more complicated and are believed to relate to power in relationships and the nature of those relationships that can be tested in situations of high pressure – in this case, watching a sports competition on television.

RESEARCH IN FOCUS

Link between watching sport and domestic violence

In June 2012, BBC News reported on research into the link between watching sport and domestic violence. According to police figures during the Euro 2012 tournament, when England beat Slovenia, nationally the rate of domestic violence reports increased by 27 per cent, compared with the corresponding days in 2009, when there were no football matches. When England lost 4–1 to Germany, domestic violence increased by 29 per cent. However, when the teams drew, there was no noticeable impact.

Statistician Professor Allan Brimicombe, an expert in domestic violence and the chair of the Crime and Justice Statistics Network, verified the figures and stated that: 'The stats are pretty conclusive. It's a definitive and significant increase.'

You can read more on this research at: www.bbc.co.uk/news/uk-england-18379093

To tackle violence in sport it is important to educate performers on how to control their emotions and to ensure that they are made aware that they are responsible for their individual actions and for fair play at all times. Governing bodies have their own disciplinary processes, which they apply to performers who have shown violence. These organising bodies are also responsible for the laws of the game and so ensuring that playing strategies that promote violence should be punished, as well as suggesting rule changes to make violence less likely (for example, changes in scrummaging and rucking in rugby).

Strategies to prevent violence

It is believed that performers should be educated to avoid violence and to control their emotions and levels of stress (see Chapter 5.4 on stress management). The performers should be more aware that their own behaviour can be copied by those who spectate and so they have a responsibility to show functional, non-violent behaviour. Sport is supposed to be about fair play, as we have seen before in this chapter; therefore, this fair-play philosophy should be promoted to performers so that they see the value in being non-violent while participating.

Violence shown by sports performers is most often dealt with by officials at the time of the incident and this can lead to punishments ranging from fines to bans and in some cases criminal investigations. The threat of such punishment is often the most powerful motive for performers to avoid violent behaviour. Governing organisations can impose further punishments on individuals or teams – for example, by docking points or by eliminating them from further competition. Effective officiating is also a strategy to avoid confrontation and violence. Many good officials recognise the signs leading up to possible violence and defuse the situation. For example, if two players are about to square up to each other in a rugby match, a quiet word from the ref about what might happen if a punch is thrown may be enough to defuse the situation. Some governing organisations can inflict punishments after the competition has finished, often through video analysis. For example, in rugby union, a 'citing commissioner' is appointed by the competition's organiser to examine evidence of foul play, which can include violent conduct.

One of the biggest influences on performers' behaviour is the coach or manager and their approach to competition. The most effective coaches promote assertion rather than aggression (see Book 1, Chapter 5.1 on aggression in sport).

Law enforcement is a powerful strategy in combating spectator violence. The current law enforcement action against football-related violence is contained in the Football Spectators Act 1989 (the FSA), as amended by the Football (Disorder) Act 2000. The FSA allows the police to arrest people identified as potential troublemakers and prevent them from travelling abroad to attend regulated football matches. The police may apply for football banning orders to prevent attendance at regulated football matches, whether played at home or abroad. A football banning order may be made on conviction for a relevant offence, or as a result of a civil application based on past conduct which has not necessarily resulted in a criminal conviction. A person made the subject of a football banning order has to comply with directions given by the Football Banning Orders Authority – to attend a police station and/or surrender a passport at specified times.

The increased use of sophisticated policing methods can help to prevent spectator violence – for example, using CCTV cameras and police hand-held video cameras. Other strategies include promoting friendship between rival supporters – for example, opposing teams' supporters playing a friendly game before the main match. Internet forums have been set up to try to establish friendship groups between rival supporters and some have tried to use social media to build bridges rather than to promote differences in opinion.

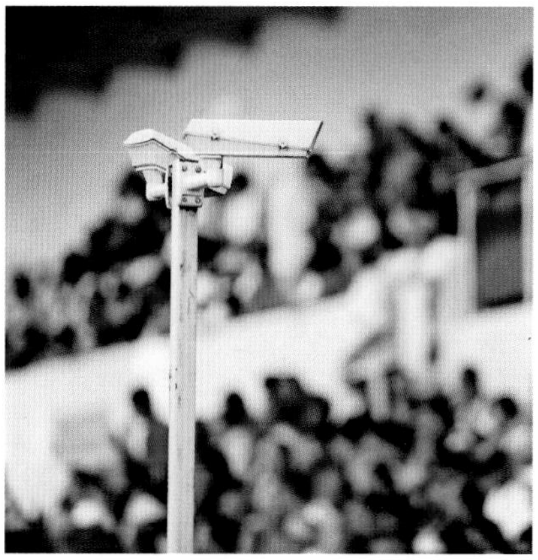

▲ Figure 6.1.6 The use of CCTV cameras can help combat violence in sport

Gambling in sport

Gambling in itself is not an example of deviant behaviour because in the UK it is legal to gamble or bet on sports events, unlike the USA where at the time of writing gambling on sports was illegal in most states. However, in this chapter we will explore **match fixing**, bribery and illegal sports betting as examples of deviance in sport.

Gambling or wagering has been a feature of sports activities over centuries of competition; indeed, there are examples of gambling in the ancient Roman Empire and more recently in Britain in the nineteenth century when wagering was closely related to events such as pedestrianism (see Chapter 6.1 in Book 1).

Sport lends itself to gambling because the outcomes of events are supposed to be unpredictable and there is an element of chance in most competitions. Many people find it exciting to watch a game or match if they are betting on the outcome or on individual aspects of the event.

Key term

Match fixing: when a sports competition is played to a completely or partly pre-determined result. This is against the law. Match fixing requires contacts to be made between corrupt players, coaches and team officials.

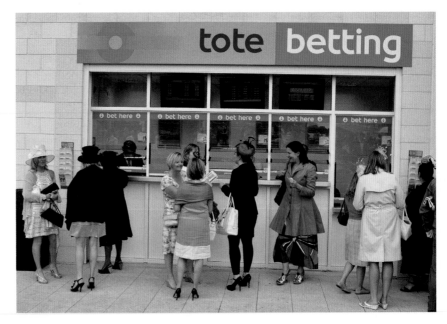

▲ Figure 6.1.7 Gambling in sport is big business

Gambling is big business worldwide and has become truly global – the growing availability of the internet has given rise to the rapid onset of gambling online. In the UK, at the time of writing, it is possible to place bets not just on the results of sports competitions but also on individual performances – for example, the number of double faults a tennis player makes, whether a player is booked by the referee in football, or how likely a batsman or batswoman is to be run out in cricket. Betting is part of the British culture and about three-quarters of the UK's adult population gambled in 2014, mostly on the National Lottery. Betting companies have moved into the sponsorship space vacated by tobacco and, to a lesser extent, alcohol. Betting companies sponsor sports clubs. A quarter of the football Premier League's clubs have gambling logos on their shirts and the Football League's 72 clubs play in competitions sponsored by Sky Bet (a betting organisation). Another betting company, William Hill, backs the Football Association. Therefore, the business of gambling is closely associated with sports organisations.

Extend your knowledge

According to Sportradar (2013), a company that analyses sports data, the amount spent on betting in the UK, including both the illegal and the legal markets, is anywhere between £435 billion and £625 billion a year. About 70 per cent of that trade has been estimated to come from trading on Association Football.

Many people enjoy gambling and are thrilled if they win a bet. Some relish the perceived excitement of gambling even if they lose – and some lose a significant amount of money. For example, West Ham footballer Matthew Etherington has been reported as losing millions of pounds because of his gambling addiction. Some sports participants and coaches have become addicted to gambling, while others have been involved in illegal gambling, bribery, match fixing and **spot fixing**. From the start of the 2014/15 football season, the FA instigated new rules regarding betting on football-related matters. Players, managers, club employees and match officials are forbidden to gamble on football events.

Key term

Spot fixing: when a specific aspect of a sports competition is illegally pre-determined – for example, a football player being sent off at a particular period of the game or a cricket bowler delivering a wide at a particular point during a game.

RESEARCH IN FOCUS

Professional footballers and cricketers are three times more likely to have gambling problems than other young men, according to research. A study (2014) conducted for the Professional Players Federation (PPF) shows 6.1 per cent of sportsmen would be classed as problem gamblers compared with 1.9 per cent in the general population of young men. The research was based on confidential questionnaires from 170 professional footballers and 176 professional cricketers.

Match fixing, bribery and illegal sports betting

Gamblers in any part of the world can place a bet on almost any professional sports event in almost any country around the world. Match fixers who have operated in Asia are now moving their operations to the rest of the world – this is where globalisation has had a negative effect on sport (see Book 1, Chapter 6.3 on globalisation). Connections are made between international 'fixers', local criminals and players or match officials.

In 2010–2011, the UK's gambling industry regulator, the Gambling Commission, investigated about 50 cases of alleged match fixing and illegal betting on British sporting events. Horse racing, football and snooker accounted for most of the match-fixing allegations in 2011. In 2000, the South Africa cricket captain Hansie Cronje admitted taking a £68,000 payment from bookmakers for providing them with match information to fix the results of games. He was banned from the sport. Jockeys are banned from betting on all horse racing, while trainers can back their own horse to win but not to lose.

IN THE NEWS

MATCH FIXING IN CRICKET

Chris Cairns, former New Zealand cricketer, was paid more than £150,000 by a pair of Indian diamond dealers in return for fixing the outcome of cricket matches, prosecutors said at his perjury trial in 2015. Allegedly Cairns had told fellow cricketers Lou Vincent and Brendon McCullum they could earn tens of thousands of dollars for fixing games, and that 'everyone was doing it'. Cairns said that since his association with match fixing his 'name had become toxic' and that it had been impossible for him to earn a living. 'I don't have any skills outside of the media,' he said. 'There was a scorched earth scenario for me. I was labouring and really just trying to make a buck.'

Study hint

It is important that you have an overview of gambling in sport and that you can recognise the financial benefits to sports organisations, as well as the considerable disadvantages of gambling addiction and the links between gambling and corruption (for instance, match fixing).

Match fixing, bribery and illegal betting are all designed to make individuals and illicit organisations a great deal of money. In the UK, a few scandals related to match fixing have hit the press, but we are relatively unscathed compared with the rest of the sporting world. This type of illegal activity is an example of deviance that is also unethical in that it is against the rules of sport and against the laws of the land.

Extend your knowledge

Incidents of match fixing, bribery and illegal sports betting involving British footballers are relatively isolated, although betting scandals go back as far as 1915 when seven players were banned after Manchester United beat Liverpool 2–0 in a match at Old Trafford where the visitors missed a penalty. An investigation was launched after complaints from bookmakers following a run of bets on the correct score line, with a goal in each half.

Nearly 50 years later, eight players were jailed for offences surrounding match fixing, including Sheffield Wednesday's 2–0 defeat by Ipswich in 1964.

A series of floodlight failures affected top-flight English matches in 1997 and later saw a businessman convicted of taking part in an Asian betting scam.

Two previous matches – West Ham v Crystal Palace and Wimbledon against Arsenal – saw the floodlights fail when the scores were level, a result favourable to a Far East betting syndicate. Nevertheless, cases of match fixing in Britain are relatively rare.

Summary

- Ethics are rules, often unwritten, that dictate your conduct. They form a system of rules that groups and societies are judged on. Deviance in sport can also be viewed as unethical. It is often as a result of the drive to win.
- Blood doping is most commonly used by endurance athletes, such as distance runners and cyclists. Anabolic steroids enable sports people to train harder and longer and often result in increased strength and aggression. Many sports performers use legal supplements to maximise training and performance in sport. The philosophy of sport is one of fair play and the taking of legal supplements is still within the bounds of acceptable fair play, whereas taking illegal substances is not deemed to be fair.
- Pressure can lead performers to use illegal means to make just enough difference to win. The influence of coaches is often underestimated because they, too, are under pressure to succeed and some strive to bask in the glory of the performers they coach. The monetary rewards are now so substantial for winning high-profile sports competition, along with the associated status and future earning capacity.
- Sports that have been associated with using illegal methods to improve performance have been tainted and have struggled to gain sponsorship. Some have lost public support – for example, cycling and weightlifting.
- WADA, the World Anti-Doping Agency, is an independent body formed by the International Olympic Committee in 1999 with the responsibility for drug testing. Governing bodies of sport all have education programmes and information about performance-enhancing drugs, their consequences and how to avoid them.
- Performers will be aggressive if they feel threatened or are frustrated by events. Some sports attract more violence than others because of the nature of the sport itself. Violence in sport cannot be isolated from society and its norms and values. Performers should be educated on how to control their emotions and to recognise that they are all responsible for their individual actions and for ensuring fair play at all times.
- Gambling is big business worldwide and is truly global since the onset of online gambling. Match fixing is when a sports competition is played to a completely or partly pre-determined result, which is against the law. Match fixing, bribery and illegal betting are all designed to make individuals and illicit organisations a great deal of money.

Check your understanding

1 What examples are there of drugs and doping in sport?

2 What are the arguments for and against the taking of legal supplements versus illegal drug taking in sport?

3 What are the reasons for elite performers to use illegal drugs?

4 What are the consequences of taking illegal performance-enhancing drugs to society, sport and performers?

5 What strategies are there to stop the use of illegal drugs and blood doping in sport?

6 What causes player violence in sport?

7 Why are some spectators violent when watching sports competitions?

8 What are the implications of violence for society, sport and performers?

9 What strategies are available to prevent player and spectator violence?

10 What examples of gambling are there related to sport?

11 What are the reasons for match fixing, bribery and illegal betting in sport?

Practice questions

1 Critically evaluate the use of legal supplements versus the taking of illegal performance-enhancing drugs in sport. (10 marks)

2 Outline the reasons why elite performers in sport use blood doping. (5 marks)

3 Discuss the consequences to performers of taking illegal performance-enhancing drugs in sport. (6 marks)

4 Describe four strategies to stop the use of illegal drugs in sport. (4 marks)

5 What are the possible causes of spectator violence in sport? (3 marks)

6 Discuss the reasons for people to gamble on sports events. What dangers are associated with gambling in sport? (10 marks)

7 Giving an example from sport, explain what is meant by match fixing. (4 marks)

6.2 Commercialisation and media

Factors leading to the commercialisation of contemporary physical activity and sport

A big factor leading to commercialisation of sport is the growing public interest in participating and watching. The commercialisation of sport over the last few decades has been dramatic, with increasing public interest globally as well as in the UK. Along with this interest come commercial opportunities to sell more goods and to use sport as a 'billboard' to show off company brands. Sport itself has benefited from this growing commercial activity and has attracted more money to increase participation, to develop facilities and to improve sporting performance.

When sport is used to advertise goods, the sport itself is promoted and the public awareness of that sport is increased, which may affect the number of people who participate or watch the sport. Each year the Wimbledon Tennis Championship is advertised well as a tournament, but it is also promoted via the advertising of companies associated with the championships. British player Andy Murray, for example, may appear on a television advert promoting a brand in question, but a by-product of this is to raise awareness of tennis as a sport. Sports organisers have used commercialism to further the causes of their sport and this has led to even more commercialisation.

The growing interest in sport is reflected in the overall increase in regular participation. Research by Sport England in 2015 shows the following:

- More people play sport at least once a week. During the year up to March 2015, 15.5 million people aged 16 years and over in England played sport at least once a week – an increase of 1.4 million since 2005/2006.
- More men play sport than women. Currently 40.6 per cent of men play sport at least once a week, compared with 30.7 per cent of women. At a younger age, men are much more likely than women to play sport, but this difference declines sharply with age.

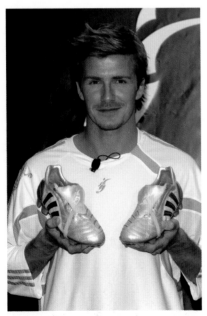

▲ Figure 6.2.1 David Beckham advertising his adidas football boots

- More younger than older people participate in sport – 54.8 per cent of 16-to-25 year olds take part in at least one sport session a week, compared with 31.9 per cent of older adults (26 plus).
- More managerial/professional workers and intermediate social groups participate regularly than manual workers and unemployed people.
- The number of both black and minority ethnic and white British adults playing sport is increasing. Slightly more people with disabilities are taking part in sport, with 17.2 per cent playing sport regularly, up from 15.1 per cent in 2005/2006.

As well as a growth in regular participation, there is growth in those who watch or spectate – see Figure 6.2.2 for growth in attendances at single sport events. The highest number of spectators for live sports events is for football in the UK, but the second highest, with more than 5.7 million people (2009 figures), is for horse racing. This rise in **spectatorship** for sports events has been an important factor that influences the commercialism of sport. More money is attracted to sports the greater their spectatorship. Businesses are aware that the more people that are involved in an activity, the more potential there will be to sell goods and services.

Activity

Using this data on sports participation, draw a graph showing the differences in participation rates.
In what ways do you think these participation rates have been affected by commercialisation in sport?

Key term

Spectatorship: the act of watching something without taking part; often related to sports spectators.

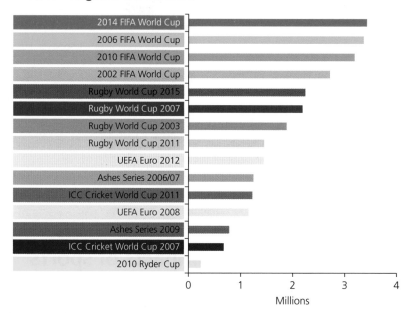

▲ Figure 6.2.2 Attendance at major single sport events has increased
Data sources: FIFA, FSMS, EY analysis

Another factor that leads to the commercialisation of sport is the growth in media interest. The fact that sports events are televised, for example, leads to more companies wishing to sponsor events and their participants. When England hosted the Rugby World Cup in 2015, the revenues from advertising for ITV, which televised the event, went up by 13 per cent. Around 2.3 million people watched the matches. For more on the effects of the media, see later in this chapter and also Part 6 in Book 1.

Greater professionalism has also led to commercialisation. Sporting professionals are more likely to attract **sponsorship** from commercial organisations. Even in a minor sport such as squash, the number of professional players has increased. For example, in 2015 there were more than 750 registered players, an increase from only a handful in the early 1980s. Professional sports participants can attract a lot of sponsorship and many

Key term

Sponsorship (in sport): to support an event, activity or person related to sport, by providing money or goods.

have significant commitments to advertise the products associated with their sponsorship. For example, in December 2014 Andy Murray signed a £15 million kit sponsorship deal over four years with the clothing firm Under Armour.

IN THE NEWS

Under his four-year sponsorship deal with the American clothing brand, Andy Murray wears Under Armour's apparel, footwear and accessories during competitions and features in marketing campaigns for the company.

The deal followed a five-year association between the British No. 1 and sportswear manufacturer adidas.

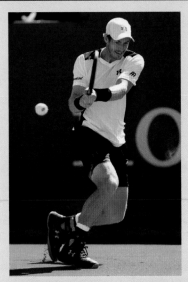

▲ Figure 6.2.3 Lucrative sponsorship deals for performers like Andy Murray have led to greater commercialisation

Study hint

When describing the factors leading to the commercialisation of contemporary physical activity and sport, comment on growth in participation and spectatorship, the increase in media interest, and the links between professional sports performers, sponsorship and advertising.

Positive and negative impacts of sports commercialisation

Commercialisation of sport has an impact on society, sports, performers and spectators. The influence of commercialism can bring many advantages, but also drawbacks. In the UK we hold a view that sport is about fair competition and that everyone has an equal chance of participating and winning in sports competitions. The sponsorship of sports performers can help to support training and competition, which enables many other people to compete on equal terms. However, whether you attract sponsorship, and how much, depends on a number of factors that may well lead to unfairness in opportunities to succeed. Some sports people are more 'marketable' than others, perhaps because of their looks, image, personality or past performance. This is a reflection of our society in which some people are more likely to succeed than others based on factors that may be other than their talent and abilities. The study of sport in this context is therefore interesting because it applies real-life social and cultural factors that exist in all walks of life.

Positive impacts

Commercialisation impacts individual sports in many positive ways. Sports can promote themselves and thus might attract more participants or spectators, which in turn can lead to increased revenues. The benefits for individual sports are often associated with bringing more money into the sport and therefore more facilities can be built and more development of the sport can take place. Sports competitions, such as leagues or tournaments, can often take place only if commercial companies invest significantly. For example, sponsorship of women's hockey by Investec, a financial products organisation, has resulted in investment in the national team, the Hockey League and 'Quicksticks', a programme introducing hockey to primary schools. As part of Investec's sponsorship, a number of events take place each year, including the Investec Women's Hockey League Finals, the Investec London Cup (a tournament created by the company) and other internationals. The sponsorship is a five-year agreement that was signed in 2011.

> **RESEARCH IN FOCUS**
>
> Commercial research shows the extent of lucrative sponsorship deals for a major FIFA tournament in 2016. The Fédération Internationale de Football Association stood to make $1.4 billion from sponsorship deals with 20 major companies during the World Cup in Brazil. That's 10 per cent more sponsorship revenue than from the previous World Cup, in South Africa.
>
> Source: Portada, 27 January 2014, latam.portada-online.com

Negative impacts

The drawbacks for individual sports include the fact that the less popular ones attract less sponsorship and therefore are unable to develop their sport to the same extent as more popular sports. Female events and those for people with disabilities may lose out on commercial investment because they are less popular and therefore would attract less media exposure for the potential sponsor.

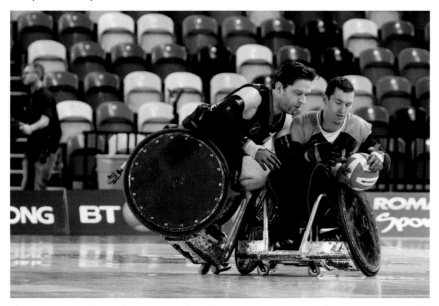

▲ Figure 6.2.4 Sports that are played and watched by a minority of people lose out on sponsorship

Businesses will sponsor all different aspects of a sports team, event or individual, including the following:

- Clothing: teams often get a shirt sponsor, for example, and individual players will get deals for clothing such as footwear. Example: O2 and England rugby shirts.
- Equipment: businesses will sponsor a player's or a team's equipment. This is usually the equipment manufacturer. Example: Wilson tennis rackets for world No. 1 Serena Williams.
- Stadiums and grounds: these may be named after the sponsor who has put money towards the building or maintenance. Example: the Emirates Stadium for Arsenal Football Club.
- Competitions: businesses sponsor competitions or leagues and then their name appears on the products related to the competition. Some competitions are named after their sponsor. Example: the Bank of Scotland Midnight League (Scottish five-a-side football) and the Barclays Premier League (football).

Performers themselves can benefit enormously from commercialism and sponsorship. They can receive kit and equipment from companies wishing them to promote their products. Commercial organisations can also fund individual athletes for accommodation and travel. Sportsmen and women with funding from business can afford to spend more time training and competing in their sport. The Badminton Company, a sports clothing and equipment company, has sponsored promising junior badminton players and provided them with rackets.

The disadvantages for individual performers include the pressure to perform well and to secure and keep sponsorship deals. This pressure to win, please sponsors and retain commercial interests has led to some deviant behaviour among performers, such as taking drugs or displaying violence. Performers are also reported to be at the beck and call of businesses that require them to promote their goods and services. Attendance at promotional events and the need to wear the appropriate sponsored clothing and use the sponsors' equipment can put a great deal of pressure on individuals in terms of time and the related anxiety of having to market these goods and services. Some performers find that they are limited in their control over their careers, with sponsors demanding that they enter particular tournaments, for example, or even having to play when injured.

Commercialism in sport can have an impact on spectators as well. Spectators at a sports event that has been supported well commercially experience a more exciting spectacle with additional entertainment, such as fireworks and light displays at a football match or spectator competitions before the match at cricket events. Commercially organised technology, such as the use of sponsored giant video screens and play-back technology, provides more information and enables a more entertaining experience for spectators. With this increase in commercialisation, some sports now have more competitions and more coverage through different types of media, which makes sport more accessible to a greater range of spectators.

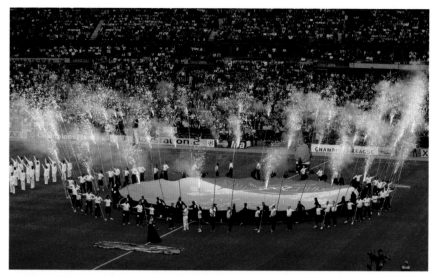

▲ Figure 6.2.5 Through commercialism, spectators experience a more exciting spectacle with added entertainment

The disadvantage for spectators is that the actual sporting action can take second place to advertisements for goods in which they may not be particularly interested. During the televised Rugby World Cup in 2015, for example, some spectators found advertising breaks to be intrusive and felt that they interrupted the flow of the event too much. During live events the advertising can become overwhelming and may spoil the viewers' enjoyment — for example, fans at football matches may have to sit through a sponsor's presentation before the match starts. When keen followers of a sport want to watch a replay on YouTube, it is usual for an advertisement to delay the start of the video and this can be detrimental to their enjoyment. Spectators may not agree with a particular company's ethics, or may be against the use of the goods being advertised — one of the 2012 Olympics sponsors was Heineken, which may not have sat well with spectators who consider alcohol to be detrimental to health. Such sponsorship might deter people from attending a sports event promoting an alcoholic beverage.

Spectators may not want their team to be associated with a particular brand — for example, Wonga (pay-day loans). Football clubs that have tried to rebrand themselves to be more commercially viable have come into conflict with their supporters. The Cardiff City owner wanted to change the team's playing shirts from blue to red (they still play in blue), and Hull City fans protested about changing the club's name to Hull Tigers when the owner felt a name change would make the club 'more marketable on the global stage' (the FA rejected the name change). Fans felt that the commercial interests of the owner outweighed their interests as spectators and supporters of the club.

Spectators for some sports events have to pay a considerable amount of money to watch — subscriptions to televised sports channels can be expensive and commercialism can be seen as doing little to make spectatorship more affordable. Commercial companies are motivated to make a profit and spectators often have to pay a high price for these profits to be realised.

Coverage of sport by the media today

Activity

Research three different ways that your chosen assessed sport is represented in the media. Identify the types of media and present the differences in audience figures for the various types of media coverage.

Media coverage linked to the globalisation of sport in the twenty-first century has been covered in Book 1, Chapter 6.2. Coverage of sport today is extensive and different types of media make sport accessible to many people. Types of media include television, print press, radio, the internet and social media, and the cinema.

In the 1980s, media coverage of sport was significantly different from the coverage today. Sports presenters became household names, such as David Vine (snooker commentator), Brian Moore (for football) and Harry Carpenter (for boxing). Note that these examples are all male because male presenters were commonplace, along with the coverage of predominantly male sport at that time. Sexism was a feature of the sports coverage, with very little attention paid to female sport. During the 1980s football hooliganism was rife and often the media were dominated by the negative aspects of sports spectators.

The fundamental changes in television coverage came in the 1990s and into the twenty-first century, with the development of satellite television. Sky spent enormous sums on securing the rights to televise football. Other television companies have followed suit to show different sports events.

Media coverage today is multi-faceted and global. In other words, different types of media are now available to most people, with the most different being online media. The media coverage is more global in terms of sports events recorded or streamed live to those who wish to subscribe or watch on free-view media. In the 1980s global events were limited to the Olympics and World Cup competitions; now many sports are accessible and more minority sports are represented, although they are still under-represented next to the major sports, as are female sport and disabled sport.

Table 6.2.1 Examples of sports coverage for different types of media

Type of media	Example of coverage (2015)	Coverage in 1980?
TV terrestrial	FA football Cup Final on BBC (and BT)	Yes
TV subscription	Football Champions League (BT)	No (Champions League started in the 1992/93 season)
TV pay per view	Test cricket (Sky)	No (not generally available in the UK until the early 1990s)
Radio sport station	Ashes Test cricket (Radio 5 live)	No (Radio 5 live started in 1994)
Radio national commercial	The Grand National (talkSPORT)	No
Newspapers	Wimbledon Tennis Championship (most daily newspapers)	Yes
Internet	Rugby Union (BT online)	No

Study hint

Make sure you are able to give examples of different sports represented in different types of media – for example, cricket commentary on Radio 5 live and pay per view boxing on Sky Sports – and how this might differ to the coverage in the 1980s.

Positive and negative effects of media on sport

On the positive side, the media raise the profile of a sport and of individual players. This can increase the numbers of people watching and participating – for example, during the Wimbledon Championships many more people go and play tennis in their spare time. Coverage of the Rugby World Cup stimulated more interest and numbers of spectators for rugby in the UK. Media coverage can also increase financial revenues in terms of sponsorship and for funding sports events and facilities.

Study hint

For more on the impacts of global media on sport, see Book 1, Chapter 6.2 on twenty-first-century sport.

RESEARCH IN FOCUS

More people tune in to sport on terrestrial television than they do on pay to view channels.

For example, the average ratings for live Test cricket on Channel 4 ranged between 1.05 million and 1.32 million each year between 2004 and 2013 (2005 excepted), while the averages for the two home series shown on Sky in 2006 were 0.23 million and 0.29 million for the Sri Lanka and Pakistan series, respectively. The media can have a positive effect on participation figures – for example, in 2006 Sky had the exclusive rights for cricket, but cricket participation rates actually rose between 2007 and 2009, and peaked at 215,500 in October 2010–October 2011 (compared with 195,200 in 2005–06).

Source: SportingSpeak, a sports policy and development blog, April 2015

Media can attract more funds for international teams and this in turn can boost sports participation. The increase in the cricket governing body's (ECB) investment in women's cricket and disability cricket ('Chance to Shine' programme) came about when the body received substantial funds from Sky. The rules of sport have been influenced by the media and this can make a sport more accessible to a wider audience – for example, rules that allow for more flowing play in hockey. Different types of media, including social media, are now more available 24/7, with live sport being broadcast from all parts of the globe. Today more minority sports or a wider range of sports are represented and there is more coverage of disability sport, such as the Paralympics.

The media can highlight and promote sensational news about sport and its participants and this can result in pressure on individual performers and their families. The media have also highlighted the negative aspects of sport, and it can be argued that this has promoted hooliganism and unrest among countries. Examples include England versus Germany competitions, such as football internationals, when the media have pictured England players wearing military helmets to promote the game, thus drawing comparisons with the Second World War.

The effects of the media on sport

The media can have an effect on individual sports, the performers and the spectators. Their positive contribution is believed to be to raise the status of individual sports and therefore to help promote the sport and increase participation and spectatorship. The media also attract more commercial interest and sponsorship.

The problem with media promotion is that some sports get left behind and therefore the dominant and traditionally male and able-bodied sports attract more coverage and more funding. The performers benefit from more exposure and can make more money and develop their careers both within their sport and outside it in the future. The main disadvantage is that the media can interfere with personal lives and can be intrusive and raise personal anxiety. Spectators get to watch more sport through extensive media coverage, but the diet they are served up can be limited to the major sports. The availability of live sport has increased, but the cost of subscriptions for access can be prohibitive. Some of the main sports events in the UK are now subscription only, so those fans who in the past would watch a football cup match on terrestrial 'free' TV now have to subscribe or pay to view.

Relationship between sport and the media

Sport is viewed as a **commodity** by commercial organisations and the media help to promote both sport and its commercial partners. The relationship between sport, sponsorship and the media is often referred to as the '**golden triangle**'.

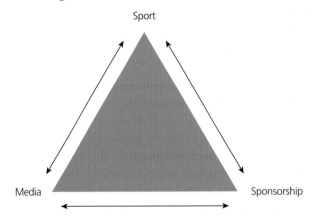

▲ Figure 6.2.6 The golden triangle – sport, sponsorship and the media

Sport, media and sponsorship are interlinked – one can influence the other. The media show sports because of the perceived needs of viewers, but there are also healthy advertising revenues. Sponsors use the media to advertise their products and they make these products even more desirable by recruiting sports stars to promote them and to be seen wearing their clothes or using their equipment. Commercial organisations pay large sums of money to advertise their products in the media, which then pay sports organisations for the rights to show their sport. Many sports get to raise their status and profile via the global media and thus can invest in the development of their elite athletes as well as help increase grassroots sports.

Key terms

Commodity: an article that can be traded. In this case sport is the article that can be sold to different media outlets or to companies that wish to associate their brand with a particular sport.

Golden triangle: the interdependence and influences of the three factors of sport, sponsorship and the media – that an aspect of one influences the other two, and vice versa.

Summary

- Sport has benefited from commercial activity and has attracted more money to increase participation, to develop facilities and to improve performance.
- In the UK sport is believed to be about fair competition and that everyone has an equal chance of participating and winning. Sponsorship of performers can help to support training and competition, which enables many to compete on equal terms.
- Some sports people are more 'marketable' than others – for example, because of their looks, image, personality or past performances. This reflects society in that some people are more likely to succeed than others based on factors that may be other than their talent and abilities.
- In the 1980s, media coverage of sport was significantly different from the coverage today. Sexism was a feature of the sports coverage at that time, with very little attention paid to female sport.
- The positive effect on sport is that the media raise the profile of a sport and of individual players. This can increase the numbers of people watching and participating in that particular sport. Media coverage can also increase the financial revenues in terms of sponsorship and funding for sports events and facilities.
- Different types of media, including social media, are now more available 24/7, with live sport being broadcast from all parts of the globe. Today more minority sports and a wider range of sports are represented, and there is more coverage of disability sport, such as the Paralympics.
- Sport, media and sponsorship are interlinked – one can influence the other. The media get healthy advertising revenues. The sponsors in business use the media to advertise their products.

Check your understanding

1 What factors lead to the commercialisation of contemporary sport?
2 What are the positive and negative impacts of commercialisation of sport on society, sports, performers and spectators?
3 What are the features of sport in the media today?
4 What are the differences between media coverage of sport in the 1980s and today?
5 What are the positive and negative effects of the media on sport?
6 What is the relationship between sport as a commodity and the media?

Practice questions

1 Explain how spectatorship has led to the commercialisation of sport. (5 marks)
2 Using examples, describe how sponsorship is a feature of contemporary sport. (4 marks)
3 Evaluate the impact of commercialisation on sport, taking into account society, individual sports and spectators. (10 marks)
4 Explain the reasons for the changes in the coverage of sport since the 1980s. (5 marks)
5 Using practical examples, outline the different types of media used today in sports coverage. (5 marks)
6 Evaluate the positive and negative effects of the media on individual sports. (6 marks)

6.3 Routes to sporting excellence in the UK

Understanding the specification

By the end of this chapter you should:

- have an understanding of the development routes from talent identification through to elite performance
- understand the role of schools, clubs and universities in contributing to elite sporting success
- know the role of UK Sport and national institutes in developing sporting excellence and high-performance sport
- be familiar with the strategies to address drop-out or failure rates from elite development programmes and at elite-level sport.

In the Autumn Statement in November 2015, the Chancellor of the Exchequer announced an increase in funding for sports excellence by 29 per cent. At a time of austerity, this was a significant increase and recognises the importance of sports success in the UK. To reach the top in sport, a considerable amount of planning is required, along with funding to pay for training, facilities, travel, equipment and coaching. A strategic view of excellence has been developed by the government and sports organisations, but the picture is a complex one because of the many agencies involved. This chapter will trace the development routes in sport and the roles that each of the agencies play in the path to sporting excellence.

From talent identification to elite performance

The identification of potential elite performers in sport has been formalised and organised by **UK Sport**. This organisation develops elite athletes by:

- identifying potential talent in sport
- supporting an athlete's lifestyle
- supporting the athlete's coaching
- supporting, through research, sports science and sports medicine, via the English Institute of Sport
- providing a 'World Class Programme' or pathway to success.

World Class Programme

The programme operates at two distinct levels:

1. Podium – supporting athletes with realistic medal-winning capabilities at the next Olympic/Paralympic Games (i.e. a maximum of four years away from the podium).

2. Podium Potential – supporting athletes whose performances suggest that they have realistic medal-winning capabilities at the subsequent Olympic and Paralympic Games (i.e. a maximum of eight years away from the podium).

Key term

UK Sport: an organisation whose aim is the development of the country's sportsmen and women (athletes). It is funded jointly by the government and the National Lottery.

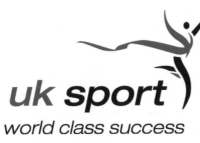

▲ Figure 6.3.1 UK Sport helps to identify and develop elite sportsmen and women

Identifying sports talent

UK Sport runs talent recruitment and talent confirmation programmes, starting with a search for those who have sporting talent, either among the general public or within sports clubs and community projects. Athletes submit an application to UK Sport, who then invite successful applicants to a 'phase 1' testing event.

Phase 1 involves physical and skills-based tests, including sprints, jumps, aerobic fitness and strength tests, depending on the sport. The selection process includes an analysis of each athlete's training and competition history. During phases 2 and 3, there is further assessment of an athlete's suitability for the sport and preparation for training and development. During these phases, sessions may include physical and medical screening, performance lifestyle workshops and psychological assessments. In the final, confirmation phase selected athletes train over 6–12 months. They are assessed continuously and rate of progress is recorded to judge their suitability for elite sport. Unsuccessful athletes are given opportunities to continue the sport through the club system.

The newly created (2016) #DiscoverYourPower initiative involves a partnership between UK Sport, the English Institute of Sport and British Cycling in the first instance, although more partnerships are planned for the future. This campaign was launched to identify future Olympic and Paralympic medal winners. These campaigns are for targeted sports such as cycling. The first campaign is aimed at young track cyclists, aged 15–21, or potential cyclists with good speed and power. It is looking for those that are competitive and have the appropriate mental approach to respond to guidance from elite coaches in a pressurised training environment. For example, there has been success in the past working with sprinters who have the speed and power that can be transferred to track cycling. #DiscoverYourPower involves a series of testing phases beginning in summer 2016, with the very best athletes joining British Cycling's National Lottery-funded World Class Programme, where they will benefit from access to world leading science, medicine and technology to help them reach their full sporting potential.

Every four years, UK Sport runs a checking system for the athletes on the programme, called the Pathway Health Check (PHC). The PHC involves discussions and shared analyses between the performance pathway team and the sport's key coaches. It takes into account, among other aspects, the athlete's progress, fitness levels achieved and whether the athlete has made a good transition between junior and senior levels. This process is a way to measure the effectiveness of the performance pathway.

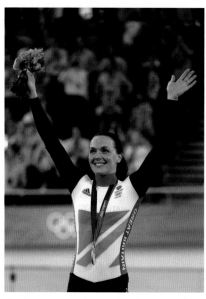

▲ Figure 6.3.2 The World Class Programme supports those athletes who have the potential to win an Olympic or Paralympic medal

IN THE NEWS

The UK Talent Team is a collaboration between UK Sport and the English Institute of Sport (EIS). It supports World Class Programmes to identify and develop talented athletes. Jayne Ellis, Paralympic Talent Scientist for the UK Talent Team, said: 'This is a fantastic opportunity for disabled people to get involved in Paralympic sport and I find it really exciting to think about the talent we could unearth through Paralympic Potential: Bring on Brazil. We are looking at potential athletes for a wide range of sports and the only criteria are you need to be fit, used to playing sport and really focused on achieving your goals. Those selected will ultimately have the chance to become part of World Class Performance Programmes within Paralympic sports here in the UK, which are regarded as being among the finest in the world.'

Source: UK Sport, November 2015

UK Sport has tried to identify sports talent through national campaigns such as 'Tall and Talented', launched to prepare potential medal winners for the 2016 Rio Olympics.

UK Sport searched for athletic men over 6 feet 3 inches and women over 5 feet 11 inches who aspired to represent Great Britain in Rio de Janeiro. The organisation wanted to identify exceptionally tall men and women who could find success in sports where height can give an athlete a real advantage, such as rowing. Coaches and sports scientists analysed each athlete's testing data – for example, from strength, endurance, power and agility tests – and sporting background, benchmarking against data collected from successful Olympians over many years.

World Class Podium and World Class Podium Potential

The World Class Programme covers all the sports in the summer and winter Olympics and Paralympics. There are two distinct levels:

1   Podium level: supporting athletes with realistic medal-winning capabilities at the next Olympic/Paralympic Games.

2   Podium Potential level: for athletes whose performances suggest that they have realistic medal-winning capabilities at the subsequent Olympic and Paralympic Games (that is, a maximum of eight years away from the podium).

Around 1,300 of the nation's leading athletes at the Podium and Podium Potential levels currently benefit from UK Sport's annual investment of around £100 million (2015 UK Sport figures). The programme works by ensuring that athletes get high-quality support via their sport's national governing body. Funding is given for coaching, training and competition support, medical, technology and scientific services delivered by the home country institutes, and access to top-quality sports facilities. It is also recognised that to succeed in the Olympics and Paralympics effectively means training and competing full-time. Therefore, UK Sport makes an 'Athlete Performance Award', which makes financial contributions towards athletes' living and sports costs via the National Lottery fund.

Case study of an athlete on the World Class Programme

Sprinter Jonnie Peacock is one of 1,300 athletes on UK Sport's World Class Programme. Jonnie lost his right leg below the knee after contracting meningococcal septicaemia at the age of five. In 2015, he was the Paralympic, World and European champion after less than ten years in the sport. It was at a talent identification day run by the British Paralympic Association in 2008 that his potential was first spotted and he was invited to train with a group of talented youngsters to accelerate his talent. He worked with well-qualified coaches and kept improving enough for London 2012. He won the T44 100 m gold in front of the 80,000 capacity crowd. Peacock is focused on improving to ensure success in Brazil 2016. He trains alongside some of the UK's brightest sprinting prospects, such as European champions Adam Gemili and James Dasaolu and European bronze medallist Harry Aikines-Aryeetey.

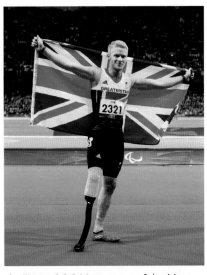

▲ Figure 6.3.3 Many successful athletes in the UK have been part of the World Class Programme, including Jonnie Peacock

The role of UK Sport in developing elite sport

The main role of UK Sport is to invest National Lottery funds and income from central government to maximise the performance of UK athletes in the Olympic and Paralympic Games and global sports events. Success is measured by the medals won and the number of medallists developed. UK Sport invests around 70 per cent of its income in two ways:

1 Central funding for sporting national governing bodies (NGBs), enabling them to operate a World Class Programme (see page 186) and ensuring that athletes have access to personal and training support to guarantee that they are prepared for world-standard competition.

2 Funding for athletes directly through the Athlete Performance Award (APA). This award, which is funded by the National Lottery, is paid directly to the athletes and contributes to their living and sporting costs.

Extend your knowledge

UK Sport – planning to support athletes' development

As well as training and development of athletes, UK Sport provides other forms of support, for example:

- development of top-class coaches
- running the talent-identification programme (see more details above)
- organisation and promotion of campaigns to fast-track future medallists into the right sports
- development of warm-weather training and acclimatisation
- ensuring that athletes have access to high-performance training facilities.

This support is typically worth around £36,000–60,000 per athlete per year at the Podium level and £23,000–40,000 per athlete at the Podium Potential level, depending on the sport.

Athlete Performance Award (APA)

The Athlete Performance Award gives money to elite athletes to help fund their living and personal sporting costs. APAs are allocated where there is the greatest financial need. UK Sport has set a maximum income threshold of £65,000 (including the APA). The level of APA received is determined by different criteria, including the level of performance an athlete has achieved and is capable of producing in the future. Athletes on Podium-level funding can currently receive APAs to the value of up to £28,000 per year (2015 figures from UK Sport).

Case study: British skeleton athletes

Over the last ten years, British skeleton has grown from a relatively unknown Olympic sport in the UK to a much better known, high-quality sport. Skeleton, named after the bony appearance of the sled, is a sliding winter sport in which a person rides a small sled down a frozen track while lying in a prone position. The World Class Programme for the sport has produced talent capable of representing Great Britain at all levels of international competition. This programme has clearly demonstrated that with systematic talent identification and development of the right athletes with proper funding, high-quality coaching, a professional management structure and investment in technical innovation, a traditionally non-winter sport nation can be successful in international competitions.

The sport received £2.1 million core Lottery funding from UK Sport between 2006 and 2010. UK Sport has also invested significant funding in the talent identification and development programme in skeleton for the last few years. High-quality sports science and medicine services have been given via the national institutes (see below). This funding has allowed British skeleton to gradually evolve its performance pathway and athlete development programmes since 2000. The overall success of this programme is clear: 13 different athletes who were on the World Class Programme won 76 medals between 2006 and 2010. Funding has given athletes living and personal training expenses, and the freedom to train full-time and be totally committed to their sport.

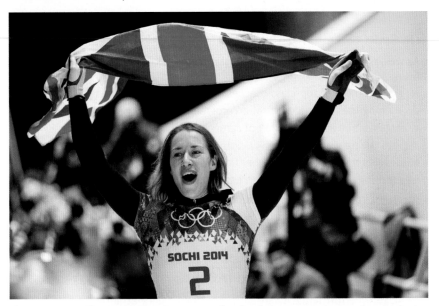

▲ Figure 6.3.4 The World Class Programme for the skeleton sport has produced talent capable of representing Great Britain, including Lizzy Yarnold

The role of the National Institutes of Sport in developing elite sport

Each country that makes up the UK has a **National Institute of Sport,** which provides sports science and technological help to elite sportsmen and women. For example, the English Sports Institute (EIS) during the period 2009–13 worked with 86 per cent of the athletes and 27 of the 29 sports that won a medal for Team GB at the 2012 Olympic and Paralympic Games. These athletes included Jessica Ennis-Hill, Mo Farah, Sir Bradley Wiggins, Sir Chris Hoy, Victoria Pendleton, Nicola Adams and Katherine Grainger.

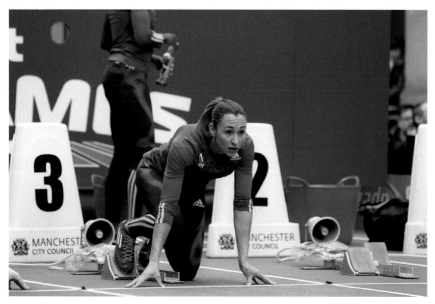

▲ Figure 6.3.5 The EIS supports the training of elite athletes

The national sports institutes work with coaches and sports administrators to help improve the performance of their athletes by giving technical support that enables them to optimise their training programmes, maximise performance in competition, and improve their health and availability to train. The EIS also has a dedicated team of sports scientists who support coaches and their athletes.

Study hint

Make sure that you can describe the role of the national institutes in developing elite athletes. Summarise their role. For example, they provide:

- science and medical staff, including physiotherapy, strength conditioning, performance nutrition and psychology, and advice on biomechanics and general lifestyle
- access to top-class facilities such as performance centres and training bases
- technology equipment that is used to test, train and support athletes and their coaches.

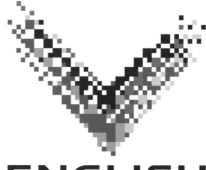

▲ Figure 6.3.6 The EIS helps to improve the performance of elite athletes

Extend your knowledge

The EIS High Performance Centres:

- Manchester
- Sheffield
- Loughborough University
- Bisham Abbey
- University of Bath
- Alexander Stadium, Birmingham
- Lee Valley Athletics Centre
- Lilleshall National Sports Centre
- National Badminton Centre, Milton Keynes.

Activity

For your chosen assessed sport, write a summary of how you might be supported to reach elite level in the UK. Refer to the government, the National Lottery, UK Sport and the National Institutes of Sport.

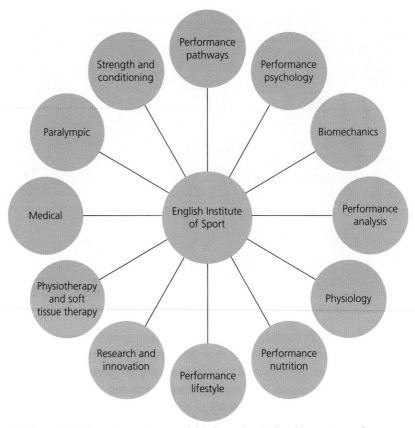

▲ Figure 6.3.7 The main services available from the EIS for elite sports performers

Strategies to address drop-out or failure rates from elite development programmes and at elite-level sport

The elite development programmes described above often lead to high-level performance and success for individual athletes and sports teams. There are, however, those who do not succeed or who drop out of the programmes because of the level of demand. Others who are not in such programmes also may find the demands of elite sport difficult to sustain and stop training and competing.

Drop-out and failure in elite sport can be a result of poor performances, injury, pressures outside the sport, such as family commitments, pressure from the media, and stress related to the financial impact of training, travelling, competing and fulfilling commitments outside of sport. For more on coping with stressors within sport, see Chapter 5.4 on stress management.

The programmes run by UK Sport via the national institutes include a lifestyle component that attempts to help athletes cope with the pressures and demands of elite sport. Lifestyle is available to all athletes on the World Class Programme. For elite athletes to maintain a performance lifestyle they must fit many aspects of their life alongside their intensive training programme. Training advisers at the EIS give athletes the necessary skills to cope with the special demands of being an elite performer and to prepare them for their life after sport.

Elite athletes are encouraged to work closely with coaches and support specialists to minimise potential concerns, conflicts and distractions, all of which can be detrimental to performance and may end a sporting career. Performance lifestyle advisers support athletes with time management, budgeting and finance, dealing with the media, sponsorship and negotiation/conflict management. Advice is also available for athletes on finding suitable jobs and deciding on a future career. This could include help with finding a job to supplement income that fits around the athlete's training demands, work placements, or planning for a career after sport.

All programmes and wider aspects of training related to elite sports performance have elements of evaluation throughout training and competition. The best sports coaches and support staff will instigate a systematic evaluation process to identify potential stressors or difficulties that an elite athlete might face and then intervene with planned strategies to try to avoid drop-out or failure in performance. These strategies can involve medical intervention and advice, physical training adaptations and psychological strategies, such as goal setting, which have been covered earlier in this book.

The role of schools, clubs and universities in contributing to elite sporting success

Schools, colleges and clubs

Schools and colleges contribute to elite sport in the UK, although their role is often less than that of Sport UK and the national institutes. Schools provide physical education for all young people and often offer extra-curricular sports activities and clubs for students who are keen to participate and for those who might excel at a particular sport. In the past schools were given funding for school–sport partnerships, but the government discontinued this as part of a cost-cutting exercise in October 2010. However, the government does supply schools with funds to support school sport and schools often use those funds to increase participation by young people and to support the development of elite sports performers. Sports organisations such as the Football Association, the England and Wales Cricket Board, the Rugby Football Union, the Lawn Tennis Association and the Premier League send coaches to primary schools in order to improve sports provision.

Schools and colleges are encouraged by organisations such as Sport England to link with community sport to increase sports participation that might lead to more young people realising their potential and becoming elite performers. Schools and colleges also provide qualifications in sport that recognise sports performance and therefore encourage elite sport – for example, GCSE Physical Education, Advanced Apprenticeships in Sport, Cambridge Nationals and Technicals in sport and, of course, the subject that you are studying, the GCE A Level in Physical Education. All these qualifications have sports performance as part of the qualification and credit is given for the quality of that performance.

Sport England

Sport England is focused on helping people and communities across the country create a sporting habit for life. It has invested more than £1 billion of National Lottery and government funding between 2012 and 2017 in organisations and projects that will:

- encourage more people to develop a sporting habit
- create more opportunities for young people to play sport
- nurture and develop talent in sport
- provide the right facilities in the right places for sports participation.

Schools and colleges often run sports teams in a wide range of activities and are involved in fixtures against other schools and colleges. This helps to develop sports talent in the UK. Both the state and private school sectors are involved in this provision, but the private sector is often in a better position to offer the required resources and funding for high-level sport.

RESEARCH IN FOCUS

The Sutton Trust (2012) is an educational charity in the UK which aims to improve social mobility and address educational disadvantage. Its research reveals that more than a third of British medal winners in the 2012 London Olympics were from private schools, which educate 7 per cent of the school population. The dominance of private schools is particularly evident in sports such as rowing, where more than half of gold medallists were privately educated, with fewer than a third coming from state comprehensives. Gold medal-winning athletes such as Jessica Ennis-Hill, Mo Farah and Greg Rutherford were state educated, as were all the boxers in the 2012 London Olympics, and all but one of the 12 medal-winning cyclists. Team GB won 65 medals, 29 of them gold.

Advanced Apprenticeships in Sport

The Advanced Level Apprenticeship in Sporting Excellence (AASE) is a sports performance programme. It provides a structured training and development route across a number of sports for talented young athletes (aged 16–19) who have a real chance of excelling in their sport, either by competing on the world stage or through securing a professional contract.

To be eligible for this apprenticeship you must also be either a professional, full-time athlete or an athlete identified by a national governing body (NGB) as 'elite' (an athlete involved in the academy environment at professional clubs). The programme length varies depending on the sport but can be from 12 months to 24 months. It is designed to directly measure the athlete's ability to plan, apply and evaluate their development in the appropriate technical, tactical, physical and psychological aspects of their sport. It also addresses wider issues such as lifestyle, career development, communication, and health and safety.

In 2015 there were more than 2,500 athletes on the AASE throughout England. More than 20 sports were involved in the AASE, including football, rugby union, rowing, boxing, tennis, swimming and disability sport, including a large number of Olympic and Commonwealth sports.

Past AASE athletes include:

- Rebecca Adlington: double Olympic Gold medallist swimmer
- Jack Wilshere: Arsenal first-team player and England international
- Sarah Stevenson: Olympic medallist taekwondo athlete
- Rachel Jennings: Ladies European Tour golfer and former England international.

Sports clubs also contribute to elite sporting success. Clubs in the UK are organised through the NGBs, which are responsible for managing their specific sport. The NGBs provide investment that supports the development of talented athletes in 43 different sports, and Sport England, through the NGBs, funds the elite programmes of netball, squash and women's rugby. Sports clubs are often in leagues and national competitions, which enable those with talent to gain competitive experience. Participants are often recognised for further development through the elite performance programmes described above. Sports clubs nurture and encourage talent, often giving financial concessions to promising young performers and providing coaching and guidance to develop their levels of sports performance. Many athletes on elite sport programmes are based within their clubs and these clubs help to deliver some of the aspects of these programmes, such as specialist coaching and physiotherapy support.

Universities

Universities play a role in contributing to sporting success in the UK. Most higher education institutions offer university sports scholarships or bursaries and although competition for these is high and the number on offer limited, those who get them have access to special support services, such as free membership of the university sports centre, physiotherapy, strength and conditioning advice or specialist coaching. Many top sporting facilities are now located at universities, so higher education is increasingly involved in the development of sporting excellence in the UK – most world-class sportsmen and women are either in the student age group or only a year or so older. At the Beijing Olympics, 58 per cent of Team GB athletes and 55 per cent of medallists had come through the university sector. In England and Wales, funding is provided through the Talented Athlete Scholarship scheme (TASS) and in Scotland, by the Winning Students scheme. They are both government-funded sports scholarship programmes, delivered through a partnership between universities and NGBs. Some universities host centres of sporting excellence, which can be linked to one of the home country sports institutes or one or more sport-specific centres.

Summary

- The identification of potential elite performers in sport has been formalised and organised by UK Sport.
- The World Class Programme operates at two distinct levels: Podium level, supporting athletes with realistic medal-winning capabilities at the next Olympic/Paralympic Games, and Podium Potential level, for athletes whose performances suggest that they have realistic medal-winning capabilities at the subsequent Olympic and Paralympic Games.
- The selection process for elite athletes involves physical and skill-based tests plus an analysis of each athlete's training and competition history.
- The final phase of talent identification is called the confirmation phase in which selected athletes from the previous phases train over a period of 6–12 months. They will be assessed continuously during this phase and their rate of progress will be recorded so that their suitability for elite sport can be judged.
- Unsuccessful athletes are given opportunities to continue the sport through the club system but are taken out of the development programme.
- The World Class Programme covers all the sports in the summer and winter Olympics and Paralympics.
- The main role of UK Sport is to invest National Lottery funds and income from central government to maximise the performance of the country's athletes in the Olympic and Paralympic Games and global sports events.
- Each country that makes up the UK has a national sports institute and provides sports science and technological help to elite sportsmen and women.
- The national sports institutes work with coaches and sports administrators to help improve the performance of their athletes by giving financial and technical support, which enables them to optimise their training programmes, maximise performance in competition, and improve their health and availability to train.
- Drop-out and failure in elite sport can be a result of poor performances, injury, pressures outside the sport, such as family commitments, pressure from the media, and stress related to having enough money to train, travel, compete and fulfil other financial commitments outside of sport.
- For elite athletes to maintain a performance lifestyle they must fit many aspects of their life alongside their intensive training programme. Training advisers at the EIS give athletes the skills to cope with the special demands of being an elite performer and to prepare them for their life after sport.
- Schools provide physical education for all young people and often offer extra-curricular sports activities and clubs for students who are keen to participate and for those who might excel at a particular sport.
- Most higher education institutions offer university sports scholarships or bursaries. Although competition for these is high and the number on offer limited, those who get them have access to special support services, such as free membership of the university sports centre.

Check your understanding

1 How is sports talent identified in the UK?

2 What are the main phases for UK Sport's talent identification?

3 How does UK Sport recognise and develop elite sport?

4 What is the role of the national institutes in developing sporting excellence?

5 What strategies can be employed to limit drop-out and failure in elite sport?

6 What role do schools and clubs play in contributing to elite sports success?

7 How do universities contribute to developing elite sport in the UK?

Practice questions

1 Explain the extent of how UK Sport and the national institutes seek to develop excellence in sport in the UK.   (10 marks)

2 Describe how sports talent is identified in the UK.   (5 marks)

3 Explain the role of universities in contributing to elite sporting success.   (4 marks)

4 Outline how schools and colleges help to develop talented young sports participants.   (3 marks)

5 Explain, using examples, the different strategies that could be used to address drop-out in elite sport.   (5 marks)

6.4 Modern technology in sport

Understanding the specification

By the end of this chapter you should:

- understand the extent to which modern technology has affected elite-level sport and general participation in sport, including increased or improved access, facilities, equipment, monitoring of exercise and safety
- be familiar with the extent to which modern technology has limited or reduced participation, including cost and the range of alternatives to physical activity and sport
- have an understanding of the extent to which modern technology has increased fair outcomes, including better timing devices, increased accountability of officials, more accurate decision-making, improved detection of foul play and improved detection of doping
- be aware of the extent to which modern technology has limited or decreased fair outcomes
- be able to know and understand the extent to which modern technology has increased entertainment, and the extent to which it has reduced or limited entertainment, including interruption and delay and reduced live attendances.

Modern technology has already advanced to a massive extent over the twenty-first century and elite athletes and those who participate in sports and physical activities have found many innovative uses for it. The ethical considerations in using such technology are now more than ever a contemporary issue to ensure fair outcomes in sport. Modern technology is used to enhance entertainment for sports spectators, yet entertainment can also be reduced by the use of technology.

Modern technology for elite-level sport and for general participation in sport

Access to sport activities has been improved through the development of technology. Modern technology has not only affected elite-level sport but also many participants representing different levels of performance.

Elite sport

Modern technology can help in assessing whether someone has the potential to be an elite athlete – for example, to test which sports discipline suits them or, in the case of rowing, whether they have the right physiological make-up to make them an elite rower. The English Institute of Sport and UK Sport both support testing for potential rowers and use modern technology to make their assessments – for example, to assess bone density and internal body fat. Modern technology can also be used to assess the health of anyone who wishes to take up a sports activity – for example, through health screening devices.

There is help for disabled performers who wish to reach the elite levels shown in the Paralympics, who are given greater accessibility to elite performance training. Others with a disability who merely wish to participate generally can benefit from modern technology. **Prosthetic** devices have been developed for athletes with a specific disability and to enable performers with disabilities to participate in sport and exercise. For example, the 'Springlite' (named after the company that manufactures prosthetic devices) prosthesis has been created for athletes who have lost a lower limb. This acts like a springboard, to aid the running action. The reduced mass of the Springlite device compared with that of the earlier wooden prosthesis is firm yet supple for sprinters, and provides some shock-absorbing properties for marathon runners.

Wheelchair devices have also benefited from modern technology, with sharply slanted back wheels for tennis players to allow the player to move quickly across the court.

Key term

Prosthetic: an artificial device that substitutes or supplements a defective part of the body.

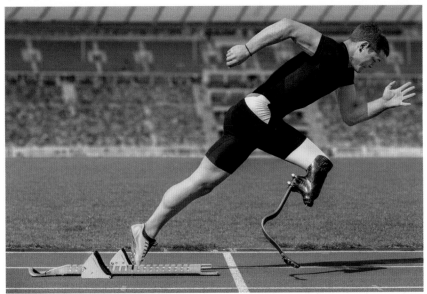

▲ Figure 6.4.1 Modern technology has helped to increase access to sport for people with disabilities

General participation

Modern technology has improved access to buildings – for example, buildings can be modified to make them wheelchair accessible and specialised equipment such as swimming pool hoists have aided pool access for elite swimmers. Modern technology has improved facilities for both able-bodied and disabled athletes. In 2009, Bisham Abbey National Sports Centre completed £2 million of elite training and rehabilitation facilities for athletes to prepare for the 2012 Olympics. The facilities included a redevelopment of a high-performance gym, with a training and agility area and a 30 m indoor track, state-of-the-art strength and conditioning machines and weights, and video-analysis equipment. It also now has more rehabilitation and medical suites. The new training and rehabilitation facilities have the latest sports science equipment that is used by rowers, canoeists and hockey players. Facilities for the elite sports competitions include different types of simulated competitive environments, such as a bobsleigh run for winter Olympic competitors and a surf simulator for elite surfers.

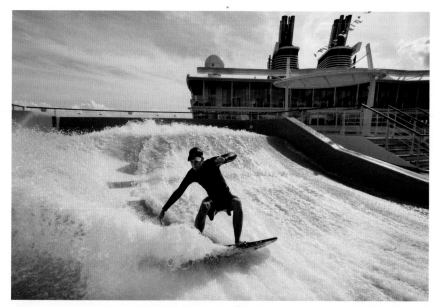

▲ Figure 6.4.2 Modern technology has enabled the development of specialist facilities, such as surf simulators

Modern technology has improved sports surfaces and artificial lighting, offering greater opportunity to play. Modern surfaces are low maintenance, therefore low cost, and allow year-round use that can help to boost participation. Surfaces have been developed to provide rebound or slip resistance and can improve shock absorption, providing optimum playing conditions for sport while giving players ease of movement and adequate protection from injury. Modern flood lighting has also allowed greater use of sports facilities at the recreational or general participation level. This has made it possible to have higher-level competition fixtures, such as day–night cricket and night-time football matches.

Modern technology has influenced the provision of equipment for elite athletes and for those who wish to participate. This equipment can help performers to train more effectively, can enable higher levels of performance, and can make training and performance safer and with minimised risk of injury. The equipment can also effectively and accurately monitor exercise rates, physiological responses and performance techniques.

The use of composite materials makes sports equipment such as rackets and protective gear lighter and more durable, enabling athletes to further improve their performance. Advances in modern technology have led to improvements in the design of sports equipment such as trainers and sports shoes and the starting blocks in athletics. For endurance athletes, altitude training is a good way of boosting fitness (see Chapter 1.2 on altitude training) by improving the body's ability to take in and transport oxygen. Modern technology has resulted in the development of the **hypoxic chamber**. This is a sealed room in which the oxygen content of the air is reduced to simulate being at altitude. Athletes then train using this room and improve their oxygen uptake.

Precision hydration techniques have used technology that was originally developed to monitor sodium loss in cystic fibrosis sufferers to assess sweat content in sports people. Electrodes coated in a special compound send a mild electrical current, which stimulates the sweat glands on the forearm.

Key terms

Hypoxic chamber: a sealed room that simulates high altitude.
Precision hydration: the monitoring of sodium loss during sweating leading to more effective replacement in the body of essential salts.

The sweat is collected and analysed. The right levels of sodium concentration for hydration during training and sports competition can then be worked out and given to the athlete in tablet form. Precision hydration has been used by numerous Premiership football clubs, national teams and sports squads.

Modern technology has also led to the development of more effective physiological testing for athletes. Laboratory-based testing is used to identify the performer's strengths and weaknesses and can monitor their progress and assess the effectiveness of their training or exercise routines. Runners, for example, can be tested on a treadmill, cyclists on a static bike, and rowers on a rowing machine. Modern technology can also be used to assess an athlete's VO_2max and lactate threshold assessment (see Chapter 1.1 on VO_2max and lactate threshold). During the 2015 Tour de France, cyclists carried miniature global positioning system (GPS) equipped computers that tracked speed, distance travelled and calories burned.

IN THE NEWS

In May 2015, Russ Thorne reported in *The Independent* on the importance of technology and engineering in the sporting world. Their impact can be seen in goal-line technology, analysis of performance data and biomechanics of body movement, even in sports clothing, such as the LZR Racer swimsuit, which reduces drag by creating a more hydrodynamic shape.

You can read the full article from *The Independent* on 18 May 2015, at www.independent.co.uk/student/shu/evolving-athletic-performance-with-the-help-of-new-sports-technologies-10218641.html

Evaluation

Technological advances in sporting equipment have added significantly to athletic performance. For example, there is some debate about whether present-day athletic achievements should be viewed with the same regard as records established in the past, when athletes were competing without the benefit of high-performance graphite tennis rackets or ultra-light running shoes.

Extend your knowledge

Modern technology and elite cyclists – wind tunnel testing

A cyclist needs to be as aerodynamic as possible, but their position needs to be comfortable while still achieving maximum power output. A wind tunnel can be used to test equipment and the body position to maximise performance. Members of the Team GB track cycling squad and triathlon team have used wind tunnel testing to enhance their performance.

Modern technology can help elite and general performers in sport avoid injury. For example, the 3D laboratory-based gait analysis allows errors in running styles to be spotted, which might cause current or future injuries. Twelve cameras record the athlete running from the side, front, back and above, and the resulting data are compared to a database of more than 3,000 uninjured runners to detect any abnormalities in running style. The coach and the athlete can then adapt the style to hopefully avoid future problems.

Personal training and performance equipment has been adapted and improved for people who wish to participate generally as well as for elite athletes. Running shoe manufacturer Asics, for example, produces specially tailored racing shoes for elite marathon runners. In some sports equipment stores, it is now common for modern technology to be used to choose the most appropriate footwear for all levels of performers, using static and dynamic foot measurements, assessment of foot shape, leg alignment and assessment of running technique.

General safety during performance is an important aspect of sport which has been improved by modern technology. For example, following the death in 2014 of Australian Test batsman Phillip Hughes when the ball struck him at the top of his neck, improvements were made in the safety standards of cricketers' helmets. The safety of performers during high-exertion activities can be monitored through the use of modern technology – for example, the introduction of ingestible computers that constantly transmit data on a player's vital functions, such as blood pressure and body temperature. For the more general participant, wearable computer devices, such as those that look like a watch strap, can monitor heart rate and the amount of activity undertaken, which can lead to more regular, efficient exercise and boost motivation to improve health and well-being.

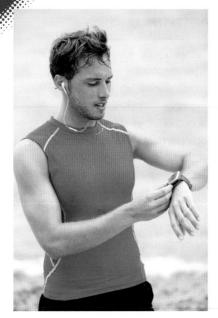
▲ Figure 6.4.3 Wearable computers can monitor heart rate and the amount of activity undertaken, which can lead to more regular, efficient exercise

When looking at the influences of modern technology on elite-level sport and for general participation, include examples of how it affects access, facilities, equipment, monitoring of exercise and safety.

Extend your knowledge

Modern technology has developed equipment so that a wider range of people can enjoy different sports activities, including those with mobility impairments:

- lightweight wheelchairs for basketball, tennis and racing
- bicycles with pedals and steering using only the rider's arms
- cross-country sit skis that allow skiers to sit down and push along the trail with tips that dig into the snow
- weights that users strap onto their wrists rather than having to hold them with their hands
- gym equipment that lets users stay in a wheelchair while using arm exercise machines
- gloves with Velcro straps that help users to hold onto an exercise machine if their grip isn't strong enough
- elastic bands that exercise muscles through resistance instead of weight
- bowling balls with hand grips to assist bowlers with limited use of their hands
- one-handed fishing rods to assist anglers who have limited mobility.

The extent to which modern technology has limited or reduced participation

We have explored many positive ways that modern technology can increase participation and performance for elite athletes as well as those who wish to participate generally. The positive aspects include improving access to the sport as well as the facilities and equipment. Modern technology helps with monitoring exercise and training levels as well as improving the performer's safety. There are, however, drawbacks with the increased use of modern technology in sport.

Cost

The development and use of modern technology is expensive and this has led to inequality for both elite and recreational performers. In developing countries, the expense of sophisticated equipment and facilities is often prohibitive. Elite athletes who are sponsored or have sufficient funding can afford the latest designs in equipment and training facilities, whereas those with limited resources may not be able to afford these and therefore are at a disadvantage. In developing countries, athletes, including those with disabilities, often lack basic equipment such as crutches, everyday wheelchairs and fundamental sports equipment. A lack of facilities or limited access to existing facilities can be problematic, and without the financial means to host large sporting events, developing countries are at a disadvantage.

The cost of modern technology is not necessarily a barrier to participation, however. At the recreational, general participation level, expensive equipment and technology are not imperative, so many people can be encouraged to participate in sport.

Range of alternatives to physical activity and sport

Modern technology, as we have seen, can increase participation in sports – for example, people with disabilities can safely participate in activities such as wheelchair basketball and skiing. However, despite the advances in technology in sport, other types of modern technology, such as computers and games consoles, can make people more sedentary and less likely to take part in sport.

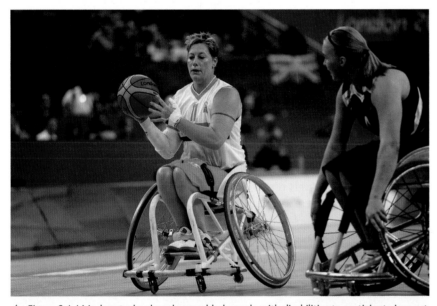

▲ Figure 6.4.4 Modern technology has enabled people with disabilities to participate in sport

Modern technology and its impact on fair outcomes in sport

Modern technology has had an influence on producing fair results or outcomes in sports competitions. Technology has resulted in gaining fairer results, but it can also be seen as hindering the likelihood of a fair result.

There are many examples of how modern technology has been used in better timing devices and in more accurate decision-making by sports competition officials, as well as in detecting foul play, including blood doping.

Most professional sports have used instant replay and other technological aids to help officials make the right decision. Rugby uses video-replay systems to check referees' decisions. Basketball referees use replay systems to make sure players are shooting within the allotted time. In international cricket, the third umpire sits off the ground with access to TV replays of certain situations, such as disputed catches, in order to advise the central umpires. The umpires out on the field are in communication with the third umpire via wireless technology.

Hawk-Eye is the name of a computer and camera system which records a ball's trajectory. It is used in tennis and cricket, and other sports are also looking at it. Although football has resisted the use of technological assistance until very recently, it is now trialling the system to assess whether a goal has been scored. Hawk-Eye uses a camera taking 600 frames a second, with the information analysed by computer. In 2015, Hawk-Eye technology was used by officials at the 2015 Rugby World Cup to improve decision-making by the television match official (TMO) and also to assist with player safety. In this case it involves video review, rather than the ball-tracking technology used in other sports.

- In Aussie rules football, an umpire review system has been implemented, with an off-field umpire in certain circumstances adjudicating on whether the ball passes over the goal line or is touched, using video evidence via multiple camera angles.
- In baseball in the USA, a challenge system was put in place in 2014 for replays to challenge certain umpiring decisions.
- In rugby union, Hawk-Eye technology was used by officials at the 2015 Rugby World Cup. Medical staff also used the video-review technology to assist with player safety by identifying possible concussion instances and behind-play incidents.
- In rugby league, officials use the video referee to help adjudicate questionable tries.

A disadvantage in using this modern technology in sport is that many officials report feeling under increasing pressure to use it more rather than make their own decisions. It also enables the media to highlight an official's mistakes during a sports competition, which can lead to judgements from the public and high levels of anxiety for the official.

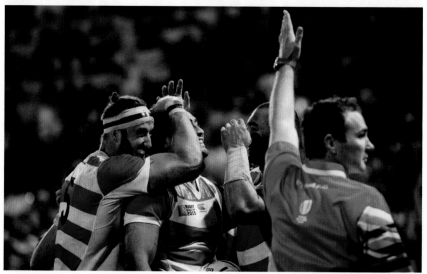

▲ Figure 6.4.5 Technology can help the media highlight an official's mistakes during a sports competition

With performance-enhancing substances and doping techniques continuously being developed by cheats, the advances in genetic technology are relevant to doping in sport. **Gene therapy** is being developed by people who want to improve sports performance. This relatively new area of medicine has proven to be clinically successful in treating several life-threatening diseases, including forms of immunodeficiency and blindness. The same methods used for therapy are potentially directly applicable to genetic enhancement, with the potential for improving athletic performance.

Key term

Gene therapy: the use of genes and genetic elements to treat human disease.

Study hint

When revising the effects of modern technology on participation and elite performance, take account of the way in which modern technology has increased fair outcomes — for example, better timing devices, increased vigilance and accountability by sports officials to make the right decisions, and improved detection of cheating. The extent to which modern technology has decreased fair outcomes should take account of limited access to such technology for some people and in some developing countries, the use of new, undetectable drugs and doping procedures, and the pressure on officials during competitions.

RESEARCH IN FOCUS

The latest research into doping in sport is being developed by Yannis Pitsiladis, a professor of sport and exercise science at the University of Brighton. Instead of looking for drugs in blood, he is searching for the 'fingerprints' that substances leave behind at the cellular level. With research supported by the WADA, Pitsiladis looks at the evidence of doping in the genetic sequence of RNA (ribonucleic acid), the partner of DNA (deoxyribonucleic acid). Professor Pitsiladis says they are developing a genetic profile, or signature, of a particular drug by taking test subjects, typically athletes not currently competing, and administering the drug to them in a controlled environment. They then analyse which genes are being affected by a drug and use that to create its genetic footprint. The advantage of this genetic approach is that it is almost impossible for this type of doping to remain undetected because of the number of genes that the drugs affect.

Source: Yannis Pitsiladis, University of Brighton, 2014

Activity

Set up a debate or discussion with other members of your class. The motion could be: 'Modern technology in sport – a dream or a nightmare?'
Select which side of the argument you wish to explore and identify the extent to which modern technology has improved elite sport, levels of participation and the likelihood of fair outcomes.

Modern technology and its impact on entertainment in sport

Sport is entertaining both for those who participate and for those who spectate. Modern technology can enhance or hinder the enjoyment of sport. It has increased the entertainment value of sport through the use of action replays and slow-motion technology. It is possible with the click of a button to rewind the action or for the television programme to show a slow-motion replay.

During live sports events there are often giant screens showing the action and also action replays, which is especially enjoyable if you have missed something or you wish to relive a successful moment for the person or team you are supporting. Modern technology also frequently involves the use of multiple camera angles so that every aspect of the performance can be viewed. A gymnast, for example, can be shown with an overhead view, from the side, back or underneath – all giving the viewer or spectator a fuller and more entertaining experience.

People who watch sport also like to assess whether officials have made the right decisions – for example, viewing many different camera angles to ascertain whether a try has been scored in rugby or whether the ball has crossed the line for a goal in hockey.

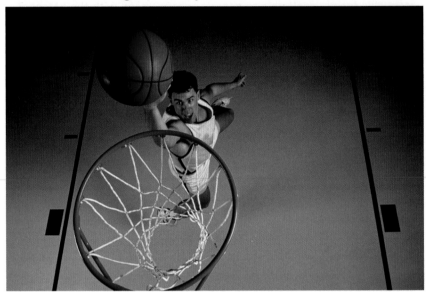

▲ Figure 6.4.6 Modern technology frequently involves the use of multiple camera angles so that every aspect of the performance can be viewed

Entertainment in sport can be enhanced through a greater understanding of what is going on, the techniques involved and the rules that should be followed. Modern technology can include different ways of analysing performance in sport so that the viewer or spectator can gain a greater insight into the event and therefore develop more interest and understanding – all of which can increase the entertainment value.

IN THE NEWS

During the Rugby World Cup in 2015, organisers were keen to reduce the time taken for TMO decisions. The England v Fiji game had stoppages of ten minutes and eight seconds for incidents referred to the TMO. John Jeffrey, World Rugby match officials selection committee chairman, stated: 'It's worth noting that just 28 per cent of stoppage time in the opening match was taken up by the TMO process, but we are committed to reducing that while not compromising on accuracy.'

You can read more on this story at: www.bbc.co.uk/sport/rugby-union/34321116

During sports **punditry**, more modern technologies are being employed, such as **motion capture analysis**, which is also used to analyse athletic performance. This involves digitally recording athletes' movements during sporting activities, the results of which can then be used for personal performance evaluation by the sports person, coaches or pundits, and for enhanced spectator entertainment.

Key terms

Punditry (in sport): typically, a knowledgeable or experienced person who, through the media, offers their opinion, guidance or commentary on a particular sport.
Motion capture analysis: the process of recording and then analysing the movement of objects or people.

However, modern technology can reduce or limit entertainment – constant interruptions, due to video playback and punditry analysis, can interfere with the flow of the event and can irritate viewers. Modern technology can break down, or there may be a delay in gathering the required information, which again can spoil the entertainment value of the event. Sport can also lose valuable revenue when spectators opt to watch instead on television or via the internet, or listen on the radio. Highlights, replays and being able to watch in the comfort of your own home, relatively inexpensively, are all reasons why modern technology may reduce live audiences at sports events.

Summary

- Modern technology is used in sport to enhance spectators' entertainment but can also reduce it.
- It can help in assessing whether someone has the potential to be an elite athlete and this improves accessibility to those who are tested and given the opportunity to develop their abilities.
- Modern technology can be used to assess the health of anyone who wishes to take up a sports activity – for example, through health screening devices.
- Prosthetic devices have been developed for athletes with a specific disability.
- Surfaces have been developed to provide rebound or slip resistance and can improve shock absorption, thus providing optimum playing conditions.
- Modern technology has influenced the provision of equipment for elite athletes and for those who wish to participate more generally. This equipment can help performers to train more effectively, can enable higher levels of performance, and can make training and performance safer, with less likelihood of injury.
- You might argue that modern technology has given an advantage to performers over rivals that do not have access to such technology. Technological advances in sporting equipment have added significantly to athletic performance.
- Modern technology has improved safety, an example being improvements in the safety standards of cricketers' helmets.
- Sports equipment and technology are an issue for developing countries and restrict participation and performance. For general participation, the expense of using sophisticated equipment and facilities is often prohibitive and may lead to a lack of motivation for participation.
- There are many examples of how modern technology has been used in better timing devices and in more accurate decision-making by competition officials, as well as improving the detection of foul play, including doping, in sport.
- A disadvantage is that many officials report feeling under increasing pressure to use modern technology rather than make their own decisions and this creates a great deal of anxiety.
- Modern technology has boosted the entertainment value of sport through the use of action replays and slow-motion technology. Different ways of analysing performance give the viewer or spectator a greater insight into the event and they therefore develop more interest and understanding, all of which can increase the entertainment value.
- Modern technology can reduce or limit entertainment. For example, constant interruptions, due to video playback and punditry analysis, can interfere with the flow of the event and can irritate viewers.

Practice questions

1 Explain, using practical examples, how modern technology has increased access for people who wish to participate generally in sport. (5 marks)

2 Evaluate the use of modern technology to improve elite performance in sport. (10 marks)

3 Outline, using practical examples, how modern technology has increased the likelihood of a fair result in sports competitions. (6 marks)

4 Entertainment in sport can be increased through sports punditry, which includes the use of modern technology. Discuss this statement using practical examples of the ways in which sports punditry uses modern technology. (8 marks)

Glossary

Abrasion: superficial damage to the skin caused by a scraping action against a surface.

Acceleration: the rate of change in velocity (m/s/s) calculated using: (final velocity − initial velocity)/time taken.

Acclimatisation: a process of gradual adaptation to a change in environment (lower pO_2 at altitude).

Achilles tendinosis: pain and deterioration of the tendon in the heel due to overuse and repetitive strain.

Acute injury: a sudden injury associated with a traumatic event.

Adenosine diphosphate (ADP): a compound formed by the removal of a phosphate bond from ATP (ATP → ADP + P + energy).

Adenosine triphosphate (ATP): a high-energy compound which is the only immediately available source of energy for muscular contraction.

Aerofoil: a streamlined shape with a curved upper surface and flat lower surface designed to give an additional lift force to a body.

Air resistance: the force that opposes the direction of motion of a body through the air.

Altitude: the height or elevation of an area above sea level.

Anaerobic: without the presence of oxygen.

Anaerobic glycolysis: the partial breakdown of glucose into pyruvic acid.

Angle of attack: the most favourable angle of release for a projectile to optimise lift force due to the Bernoulli principle.

Angular analogue of Newton's first law of motion: the angular equivalent of Newton's first law of motion which states: a rotating body will continue to turn about its axis of rotation with constant angular momentum unless acted upon by an eccentric force or external torque.

Angular momentum: the quantity of angular motion possessed by a body.

Angular motion: movement of a body or part of a body in a circular path about an axis of rotation.

Angular velocity: the rate of change in angular displacement measured in radians per second (rate of spin).

Arthroscopy: a minimally invasive surgical procedure to examine and repair damage within a joint.

ATPase: an enzyme that catalyses the breakdown of ATP.

Barometric pressure: the pressure exerted by the earth's atmosphere at any given point.

Bernoulli principle: creation of an additional lift force on a projectile in flight resulting from Bernoulli's conclusion that the higher the velocity of air flow, the lower the surrounding pressure.

Blister: friction forming separation of layers of skin where a pocket of fluid forms.

Blood doping: defined by WADA (World Anti-Doping Agency) as the misuse of techniques and/or substances to increases one's red blood cell count.

Bone spurs: outgrowths of bone into a joint causing pain and restricted movement.

Buffering capacity: the ability of hydrogen carbonate ions (buffers) to neutralise the effects of lactic acid in the blood stream.

Cardiovascular drift: upward drift in heart rate during sustained steady-state activity associated with an increase in body temperature.

Centre of mass: the point at which a body is balanced in all directions. The point from which weight appears to act.

Chronic injury: a slowly developed injury associated with overuse.

Chunking: different pieces of information can be grouped (or chunked) together and then remembered as one piece of information.

Cold therapy or cryotherapy: applying ice or cold to an injury or after exercise for a therapeutic effect, such as reduced swelling.

Commodity: an article that can be traded. In this case sport is the article that can be sold to different media outlets or to companies who wish to associate their brand with a particular sport.

Concussion: a traumatic brain injury resulting in a disturbance of brain function.

Concussion six Rs: protocol for recognition of concussion: recognise, remove, refer, rest, recover and return.

Conservation of angular momentum: angular momentum is a conserved quantity which remains constant unless an external eccentric force or torque is applied.

Contingency approach: the success of leadership traits is determined by situational factors.

Contrast therapy: the use of alternate cold and heat for a therapeutic effect, such as increased blood flow.

Controllability: whether attributions are under the control of the performer or under the control of others.

Coupled reaction: where the products of one reaction are used in another reaction.

Creatine kinase: an enzyme which catalyses the breakdown of phosphocreatine (PC).

Deceleration: the rate of change (decrease or negative) in velocity (m/s/s).

Dehydration: loss of water in body tissues largely caused by sweating.

Deindividuation: when you lose your sense of being an individual; this can cause violent behaviour.

Delayed onset muscle soreness (DOMS): pain and stiffness felt in the muscle which peaks 24–72 hours after exercise, associated with eccentric muscle contractions.

Deviance: unacceptable behaviour within a culture. Any behaviour which differs from the perceived social or legal norm is seen as deviant.

Diffusion: the movement of a gas across a membrane down a gradient from an area of high pressure (or concentration) to an area of low pressure (or concentration).

Direct force: a force applied through the centre of mass resulting in linear motion.

Dislocation: the displacement of one bone from another out of their original position.

Displacement: the shortest straight-line route from start to finish positions (m).

Distance: the total length covered from start to finish positions (m).

Distance/time graph: a visual representation of the distance travelled plotted against the time taken.

Drag: the force that opposes the direction of motion of a body through the water.

Eccentric force: a force applied outside the centre of mass resulting in angular motion.

Electron transport chain (ETC): the third stage of the aerobic system producing energy to resynthesise 34 ATP in the mitochondrial cristae.

Endothermic reaction: a chemical reaction which absorbs energy.

Energy continuum: the relative contribution of each energy system to overall energy production depending on intensity and duration.

Enzyme: biological catalyst which increases the speed of chemical reactions.

Ergogenic aids: external influences that are intended to improve athletic performance.

Erythropoietin: a naturally produced hormone responsible for the production of red blood cells.

Ethics: rules that dictate an individual's conduct. They form a system of rules that groups and societies are judged on. An ethic in sport would be that athletes stick to the spirit of the rules of the game.

Excess post-exercise oxygen consumption (EPOC): the volume of oxygen consumed post exercise to return the body to a pre-exercise state.

Exothermic reaction: a chemical reaction which releases energy.

Extrinsic injury risk factor: an injury risk or force from outside of the body.

Fast alactacid recovery: the initial fast stage of EPOC where oxygen consumed within three minutes resaturates haemoglobin and myoglobin stores and provides the energy for ATP and PC resynthesis.

Fracture: a partial or complete break in a bone due to an excessive force that overcomes the bone's potential to flex.

Gene therapy: the use of genes and genetic elements to treat human disease.

Gluconeogenesis/glyconeogenesis: the formation of glucose/glycogen from substrates such as pyruvic acid.

Golden triangle: the interdependence and influences of the three factors of sport, sponsorship and the media – that an aspect of one influences the other two, and vice versa.

Gradient (of graph): the slope of a graph at a particular moment in time. Gradient = change in y axis/change in x axis.

Haematoma: localised congealed bleeding from the ruptured blood vessels.

Hard tissue injury: damage to the bone, joint or cartilage, including fractures and dislocations.

Heat therapy: applying heat to an area before training for a therapeutic effect, such as increased blood flow.

Hook: a type of sidespin used to deviate a projectile's flight path to the left.

Humidity: the amount of water vapour in the atmospheric air.

Hyperthermia: significantly raised core body temperature.

Hypoxic chamber: a sealed room that simulates high altitude.

Intermittent exercise: activity where the intensity alternates, either during interval training between work and relief intervals or during a game with breaks of play and changes in intensity.

Intrinsic injury risk factor: an injury risk or force from inside of the body.

Kreb's cycle: the second stage of the aerobic system producing energy to resynthesise 2 ATP in the mitochondrial matrix.

Lactate dehydrogenase (LDH): an enzyme which catalyses the conversion of pyruvic acid into lactic acid.

Lift force: an additional force created by a pressure gradient forming on opposing surfaces of an aerofoil moving through a fluid.

Linear motion: movement of a body in a straight or curved line, where all parts move the same distance, in the same direction over the same time.

Lipase: an enzyme which catalyses the breakdown of triglycerides into free fatty acids (FFAs) and glycerol.

Magnus effect: creation of an additional Magnus force on a spinning projectile which deviates the flight path.

Magnus force: a force created from a pressure gradient on opposing surfaces of a spinning body moving through the air.

Massage therapy: a physical therapy used for injury prevention and soft tissue injury treatment.

Match fixing: a sports competition is played to a completely or partly pre-determined result which is against the law. Match fixing requires contacts to be made between corrupt players, coaches and team officials.

Memory trace: brain cells retain or store information.

Menisci: a tough disc of fibrocartilage in the knee joint which stabilises and absorbs shock during weight-bearing activity.

Mental rehearsal: the technique of forming a mental image of the skill or event that you are about to perform.

Metabolism: the chemical processes that occur within a cell to maintain life. Some substances are broken down to provide energy while others are resynthesised to store energy.

Mindfulness: a therapeutic technique, often involving meditation, with the individual taking into account the present. It concerns our environmental awareness and our relationships with others at a particular point in time.

Mitochondria: a structure within the cell where aerobic respiration and energy production occurs.

Mole: a unit of substance quantity.

Moment of inertia: the resistance of a body to change its state of angular motion or rotation.

Motion capture analysis: the process of recording and then analysing the movement of objects or people (in sport).

Myoglobin: a red protein in the muscle cell responsible for carrying and storing oxygen.

National Institutes of Sport: the national sports institutes that work with coaches and sports administrators to help improve the performance of their athletes.

Non-parabolic flight path: a flight path asymmetrical about its highest point caused by the dominant force of air resistance on the projectile.

Non-steroid anti-inflammatory drugs (NSAIDS): medication taken to reduce inflammation, temperature and pain following injury.

OBLA: the onset of blood lactate accumulation. The point at which blood lactate levels significantly rise and fatigue sets in.

Osteoarthritis: degeneration of articular cartilage from the bone surfaces within a joint causing pain and restricted movement.

Oxygen deficit: the volume of oxygen that would be required to complete an activity entirely aerobically.

Parabola: a uniform curve symmetrical about its highest point.

Parabolic flight path: a flight path symmetrical about its highest point caused by the dominant weight force of a projectile.

Parallelogram of forces: a parallelogram illustrating the theory that a diagonal drawn from the point where forces are represented in size and direction shows the resultant force acting.

Partial pressure: the pressure exerted by an individual gas held in a mixture of gases.

Phosphocreatine: a high energy compound stored in the muscle cell and broken down for ATP resynthesis.

Phosphofructokinase (PFK): an enzyme which catalyses the breakdown of glucose (glycolysis).

Physiotherapy: physical treatment of injuries and disease using methods such as mobilisation, massage, exercise therapy and postural training.

Precision hydration: the monitoring of sodium loss during sweating leading to more effective replacement in the body of essential salts.

PRICE: protocol for the treatment of acute injuries: protection, rest, ice, compression and elevation.

Principal axis of rotation: an imaginary line that passes through the centre of mass about which a body rotates: longitudinal, transverse and frontal axis.

Projectile: a body which is launched into the air losing contact with the ground surface, such as a discus or long jumper.

Projectile motion: movement of a body through the air following a curved flight path under the force of gravity.

Prosthetic: an artificial device that substitutes or supplements a defective part of the body.

Punditry (in sport): typically, a knowledgeable or experienced person who, through the media, offers their opinion, guidance or commentary on a particular sport.

Radian(rad): a unit of measurement of the angle through which a body rotates. $360^0 = 2\pi$ radians, 1 radian = 57.3^0.

Rehabilitation: the process of restoring full physical function after an injury has occurred.

Resultant force: the sum of all forces acting on a body or the net force acting on the projectile.

Rupture: a complete tear of a muscle, tendon or ligament.

SALTAPS: protocol for the assessment of a sporting injury: stop, ask, look, touch, active movement, passive movement and strength testing.

Sarcoplasm: the cytoplasm or fluid within the muscle cell which holds stores of phosphocreatine, glycogen and myoglobin.

Selective attention: relevant information is filtered through into the short-term memory and irrelevant information is lost or forgotten.

Self-efficacy: the self-confidence we have in specific situations.

Self-esteem: the feeling of self-worth that determines how valuable and competent we feel.

Self-serving bias: a person's tendency to attribute his or her failure to external reasons. 'I lost the badminton match because the floor was too slippy' – an excuse to explain their poor performance.

Shin splints/medial tibial stress syndrome (MTSS): chronic shin pain due to the inflammation of muscles and stress on the tendon attachments to the surface of the tibia.

Slice: a type of sidespin used to deviate a projectile's flight path to the right.

Soft tissue injury: damage to the skin, muscle, tendon or ligament including tears, strains and sprains.

Spectatorship: the act of watching something without taking part; often related to sports spectators.

Speed: the rate of change in distance (m/s) calculated using: distance/time taken.

Speed/time graph: a visual representation of the speed of motion plotted against the time taken.

Sponsorship (in sport): to support an event, activity or person related to sport, by providing money or goods.

Sports confidence: the belief or degree of certainty individuals possess about their ability to be successful in sport.

Spot fixing: a specific aspect of a sports competition is illegally pre-determined – for example, a football player being sent off at a particular period of the game or a cricket bowler delivering a wide at a particular point during a game.

Sprain: overstretch or a tear in the ligament which connects bone to bone.

State anxiety: anxiety that is felt in a particular situation (also known as 'A-state'). There are two types of state anxiety:

somatic – the body's response (e.g. tension, increase in pulse rate); cognitive – psychological worry over the situation.

Strain: overstretch or a tear in the muscle or tendon which connects muscle to bone.

Streamlining: the creation of smooth air flow around an aerodynamic shape.

Stress: stress in sport is more often linked to negative feelings and can be seen as a psychological state produced by perceived physiological and psychological forces acting on our sense of well-being.

Stress fracture: a tiny crack in the surface of a bone caused by overuse.

Subjective perceptions of outcome: how someone interprets their performance in sport.

Subluxation: an incomplete or partial dislocation.

Tendinosis: the deterioration of a tendon in response to chronic overuse and repetitive strain.

Tennis elbow: tendon pain in the forearm due to chronic overuse and repetitive strain.

Thermoreceptors: sensory receptors which sense a change in temperature and relay information to the brain.

Thermoregulation: the process of maintaining internal core temperature.

Threshold: the point an athlete's predominant energy production moves from one energy system to another.

Torque: a measure of the turning (rotational or eccentric) force applied to a body.

Trait anxiety: a trait that is enduring in an individual (also known as 'A-trait'). A performer with high trait anxiety has the predisposition or the potential to react to situations with apprehension.

UK Sport: an organisation whose aim is the development of UK's sportsmen and women (athletes) and is funded jointly by the UK government and the National Lottery.

Velocity: the rate of change in displacement (m/s) calculated using displacement/time taken.

Velocity/time graph: a visual representation of the velocity of motion plotted against the time taken.

Vicarious learning: the person observes that a reward is given to another for certain behaviours and learns to emulate that same behaviour.

Violence: intense physical force that is directed towards harming another individual or groups of individuals that can cause injury or death.

VO_2max: maximum volume of oxygen inspired, transported and utilised per minute during exhaustive exercise.

Work to relief ratio: the volume of relief in relation to the volume of work performed.

Index

Page numbers in *italics* refer to illustrations; page numbers in **bold** refer to terms covered in Extend your knowledge sections.

213